Heartburn

How to Adopt an Effettive Acid Reflux Diet to Stop Your Heartburn Problems

(Effective Way to Prevent and Heal Chronic Gastrointestinal Disorders)

Mark Burrus

Published By **Simon Dough**

Mark Burrus

All Rights Reserved

Heartburn: How to Adopt an Effettive Acid Reflux Diet to Stop Your Heartburn Problems (Effective Way to Prevent and Heal Chronic Gastrointestinal Disorders)

ISBN   978-1-998769-79-7

Legal & Disclaimer

Table of contents

Introduction

Gastroesophageal reflux disease (GERD) or gastro-oesophageal reflux disease (GORD) is an ongoing condition wherein stomach items and corrosive ascent up into the throat, bringing about side effects as well as complications. Symptoms remember the flavor of corrosive for the rear of the mouth, indigestion, terrible breath, chest torment, disgorging, breathing issues, and eroding of the teeth. Difficulties incorporate esophagitis, esophageal injury, and Barrett's esophagus.

Acid reflux, otherwise called pyrosis, cardialgia or corrosive indigestion, is a consuming sensation in the focal chest or upper focal abdomen. Heartburn is typically because of spewing forth of gastric corrosive (gastric reflux) into the throat. It is the significant side effect of gastroesophageal reflux disease (GERD).

The term acid reflux incorporates indigestion alongside various other symptoms. Indigestion is some of the time characterized as a blend of epigastric torment and heartburn. Heartburn is ordinarily utilized reciprocally with gastroesophageal reflux disease (GERD) as opposed to simply to depict a side effect of consuming in one's chest.

Reflux is a refining strategy including the buildup of fumes and the arrival of this condensate to the framework from which it started.

15% (North American and European populations)

Risk factors incorporate heftiness, pregnancy, smoking, hiatal hernia, and taking specific meds. Drugs that might cause or demolish the disease incorporate benzodiazepines, calcium channel blockers, tricyclic antidepressants, NSAIDs, and certain asthma prescriptions. Heartburn is because of unfortunate conclusion of the lower esophageal sphincter, which is at the intersection between the stomach and the throat. Finding among the people who don't improve with less difficult measures might include gastroscopy, upper GI series, esophageal pH observing, or esophageal manometry.

In the Western world, somewhere in the range of 10 and 20% of the populace is impacted by GERD. Occasional gastroesophageal reflux without irksome side effects or entanglements is much more common. The exemplary side effects of GERD were first portrayed in 1925, when Friedenwald and Feldman remarked on indigestion and its conceivable relationship to a hiatal hernia. In 1934 gastroenterologist Asher Winkelstein depicted reflux and credited the side effects to stomach acid.

Chapter 1: What Is Heartburn?

Heartburn is a condition that involves the body's upper digestive system. It is described as an uncomfortable and burning sensation behind the breastbone. Contrary to what other people think, this condition doesn't affect the heart at all even if the pain starts in the chest area before travelling to the neck, throat and jaw areas. It is also mistaken as the beginning of a heart attack but the symptoms are different.

Heartburn occurs when the acid produced in a person's stomach seeps out and is forced up to the esophagus. This leads to a bitter and sour taste in the back of the mouth and pain in the chest. Heartburn usually worsens when a person is lying down or bending over.

Understanding Heartburn

The esophagus is a tube that connects the mouth to the stomach. Normally, stomach acid should not reflux upward to the esophagus. The stomach possesses a thick protective mucus layer to prevent digestive acid from burning its lining. Although the esophagus doesn't have this type of protective lining, it has a sphincter muscle. This muscle opens up to allow food and liquids to continuously flow into the stomach and then immediately closes to stop acid and food from going back up.

When the esophagus' sphincter muscle becomes relaxed, weak or overwhelmed, it cannot stop the contents of the stomach from coming back up to the esophagus. When this happens, heartburn starts. This condition is known as Gastroesophageal Reflux Disease or GERD. If the bouts of heartburn are minimal and usually occur only after eating a hefty meal or downing copious amounts of alcohol, then that heartburn is due to plain acid reflux.

Heartburn Complications

Although heartburn is common, complications can still arise if more serious symptoms are left ignored. A frequent occurrence of heartburn means that a person's esophagus is constantly being irritated and inflamed by stomach acid. Over time, the acid can break down the tissue in the esophagus and could lead to ulcers and even excessive bleeding. The constant occurrence of heartburn can also increase risk of esophageal cancer.

Chapter 2: Causes Of Heartburn

Heartburn is a common problem for many people. Heartburn is a symptom of gastroesophageal reflux disease also known as GERD. It is usually a result of acid refluxing back into the esophagus.

The causes of heartburn are not the same for everyone. What could cause heartburn in one person could be totally different from the cause of heartburn in another person. In some circumstances a person could suffer from heartburn as a result of one cause while in other cases the condition could be caused by multiple factors.

After the stomach has digested food, the stomach juices can at times flow back up and into the esophagus. When this happens the walls of esophagus get irritated resulting in a burning sensation especially near the heart. Listed below are many of the causes of heartburn.

Hiatal Hernia

Heartburn could be caused by a hiatal hernia. Conversely, the hernia could be caused by heartburn. The two have a known link, but it is quite typical to have one and not the other. For people suffering from a hiatal hernia, a small portion of the upper region of the stomach that is linked to the esophagus is shoved up through the diaphragm. The diaphragm is a muscle that acts as a divider between the abdominal area and the chest. If an individual suffers from this type of hernia, the entry from the esophagus to the stomach is no longer in the right place. When this condition occurs, reflux is much more likely, and that means heartburn is much more likely.

Certain Types of Food

Some of the common food types we eat everyday could be a potential cause of heartburn. These foods stimulate a high secretion of stomach acid and this creates the conditions for heartburn.

Some over-the-counter drugs also are known to cause heartburn. Aspirin is an over-the-counter drug that may cause heartburn.

Overeating may also cause heartburn due to the creation of too much pressure within the stomach. The food and drink that could cause heartburn include alcohol, acidic juices such as orange juice and pineapple juice, acidic foods such as tomatoes, oranges, and grapefruit, chocolate, caffeine, foods high in fats and oils, and carbonated beverages.

Pregnancy

The increased pressure within the abdominal cavity may cause a woman to have heartburn.

Obesity

An overweight individual is more likely to suffer from heartburn. Being overweight is a condition that may contribute to getting heartburn due to increased pressure in the abdomen.

Gastroparesis

This is a condition where the stomach can't empty in a normal manner. The food sits for too long in the stomach and high acidic levels build-up resulting in heartburn.

Smoking

Tobacco weakens the lower esophageal sphincter. The smoke from cigarettes weakens the lower esophageal sphincter as it passes from the lungs into the blood. Smoking tends to adversely affect the working of the lower esophageal sphincter, making it relax; allowing acid reflux into the esophagus, bringing on heartburn.

Tea, Coffee and Other Caffeinated Drinks

Caffeine plays a big role in relaxing the lower esophageal sphincter which results in the stomach contents refluxing into the esophagus, resulting in heartburn.

Fried and Fatty Foods

Since these kinds of foods are slow to digest, the food ends up staying in the stomach longer than it should. When the food stays in the stomach longer than it should it exerts longer term pressure on the stomach and thus on the LES (lower esophageal sphincter). This results in the stomach contents refluxing.

Alcohol

Alcohol plays quite a big role in relaxing the lower esophageal sphincter. This allows the refluxing of stomach contents into the esophagus. This then results in heartburn. Alcohol also plays a huge role when it comes to stomach acid production. Stomach acid is also a common cause of heartburn.

Large meals

When someone eats a large meal, the resulting full stomach tends to exert extra pressure on the lower esophageal sphincter, which results in the stomach contents refluxing - causing heartburn.

Chocolate

Chocolate contains an element called theobromine. Theobromine is naturally found in tea, coffee and cocoa plants. It relaxes the lower esophageal sphincter. This results in stomach acid squirting into the esophagus, resulting in heartburn.

Eating 2 to 3 Hours Before Bedtime

Sleeping on a full stomach can result in the stomach contents pressing against the lower esophageal sphincter. This can result in the stomach contents refluxing and causing heartburn.

Wearing Tightly Fitting Clothes

As funny as this cause sounds, clothes that tightly fit around the abdomen tend to squeeze the stomach, which in turn presses against the lower esophageal sphincter. This results in the stomach contents refluxing to cause heartburn.

There are other foods that relax the lower esophageal sphincter. This results in the stomach contents refluxing to cause heartburn. The foods that are most likely to do this include citrus fruits, citrus juices, tomatoes as well as tomato-based products.

Chapter 3: Heartburn Triggers And Diagnosis

The frequency of heartburn varies from person to person. For some individuals, heartburn happens very rarely. But there are other people who experience it on a daily basis. Certain triggers can contribute to the repeated occurrence of heartburn.

1) Eating large portions of food: Eating too fast and swallowing food without chewing properly also increases the risk of heartburn.

2) Different drinks: This includes coffee, tea, carbonated drinks, citrus juices and alcohol.

3) Certain types of food: Spices, pepper, onions, garlic, tomatoes, citrus fruits, and fatty food cause heartburn.

4) Obesity and excess body weight

5) Smoking and being exposed to cigarette smoke

6) Wearing overly tight-fitting clothes and belts

7) Intense stress

8) Various actions and movements: running, swimming, bending over and lying down (especially after eating a full meal) triggers heartburn and may also exacerbate pain.

9) Pregnancy: Pregnant women are quite prone to different aches and pains due to the increased pressure in their abdomens. Heartburn is one of them.

10) Hiatal hernia: This is a condition wherein a part of a person's stomach protrudes or pushes through the esophageal haitus and lies in the chest cavity instead of in the abdominal cavity.

11) Esophagus-related diseases: People affected with sarcoidosis and scleroderma often experience heartburn as it is one of the symptoms of these diseases.

12) Certain medications: Taking aspirin, antibiotics, osteoporosis and blood pressure drugs, ibuprofen, and Naproxen causes heartburn in some people.

Tracking Triggers

Heartburn is a truly annoying and uncomfortable condition. It adversely affects your daily activities, interrupts a night's sleep, and limits your food choices. Fortunately, you can help prevent future heartburn episodes by keeping track of what you eat and what you do.

Keeping a record of what you eat and drink can help you find the food that is causing the condition for you. Your heartburn diary should contain comprehensive information including:

1. The type of food and drink that you consumed and when

2. Type, time, and duration of exercise

3. Medicine you take, dosage, and time of intake

4. Also, note any pain that you experience. Describe it as vividly as you can and specify when it started (after eating chocolate, after breakfast, etc.) and how long it lasts.

With proper medication and trigger tracking, you can determine the causes of your heartburn attacks and prevent future ones. The noted frequency, severity, and duration of these attacks can help your doctor diagnose underlying medical conditions, if any.

Heartburn Diagnosis

It is best to see your doctor if you experience heartburn frequently, or if the episodes are getting longer or if the pain is getting worse each time. After a brief medical history interview and physical examination, your doctor will conduct a variety of tests to find out if your heartburn is a symptom of a more serious medical condition. Some of the tests your doctor may undertake include:

1. Upper digestive system X-Ray – also known as an upper GI series and barium swallow. You will be asked to swallow a thick liquid before the X-ray procedure. The liquid will coat and fill the lining of the digestive tract to allow the specialist to see the actual silhouette of your upper intestine, stomach and esophagus. Any abnormal change in their shape and condition can signify an underlying condition.

2. Ambulatory pH probe test – this particular test will measure the amount of acid in your esophagus. The probe test involves the insertion of a catheter through your nose and into your esophagus.

3. Esophageal motility test – This test is done to determine the pressure and movement in your esophagus. The esophageal motility test also requires placing a tube in the nose and through the esophagus.

4. Endoscopy – An endoscope is a thin, flexible tube with a camera and light on its

end. It is inserted in your throat and straight down to the esophagus and stomach. The image produced by the endoscope permits a visual examination to determine any abnormal activity or growth.

Once all the tests are done, your doctor can proceed with the appropriate treatments to treat and oftentimes cure your heartburn.

Chapter 4: Heartburn Treatments

There are many treatments available to get relief from heartburn. You have a choice between prescription drugs and over-the-counter ones. These medications can either prevent heartburn from happening or relieve heartburn-related symptoms as they occur.

Prescription Drugs

1. Promotility Agents – These drugs speed up digestion which prevents acid from staying in the stomach too long, reducing acid reflux occurrences.

2. Proton pump inhibitors or PPIs – Your doctor can prescribe proton pump inhibitors if your condition is severe. These drugs effectively stop acid production to reduce the frequency of your heartburn.

Over-the-Counter Medications

1. Antacids – This is the most common heartburn treatment sold in drugstores. Because it effectively neutralizes stomach acid, antacids are used to relieve indigestion, sour stomach, and sometimes even aid in treating an ulcer.

2. Acid blockers – Acid blockers minimize acid production in the stomach to prevent heartburn, sour stomach, and acid indigestion.

3. H2 Antagonists – These drugs effectively block histamine receptors in your stomach to prevent excessive acid production. Sold in pharmacies to individuals over 16 years old, H2 Antagonists are not suitable for people with kidney or liver problems.

Like all types of drugs, these heartburn medications are not without side effects. Make sure to take these medicines according to your doctor's orders or the package instructions. You may need to take these medications only during a heartburn episode or on a daily basis for several weeks or months.

Heartburn Surgery

If your heartburn symptoms are severe and are not alleviated by any of the available medications, your doctor may recommend invasive heartburn surgery. Surgery is also indicated if you are diagnosed with GERD, Barrett's esophagus, or chronic esophagus inflammation.

Fundoplication is the type of surgery performed to ease heartburn symptoms. In this surgery, the topmost part of your stomach will be wrapped around the base of your esophagus. This will help strengthen the sphincter muscles to prevent acid reflux. After surgery, you may need to take some medication to control heartburn symptoms.

Undergoing fundoplication may make it hard for you to swallow and cause you to feel constantly bloated. Rare and serious side effects include heart problems and infections.

Endoscopic Treatments

A fairly new innovation in the medical community, endoscopic treatment is quite different from fundoplication because it does not require any incisions. To conduct the procedure, a thin, flexible tube is inserted in the throat and through the esophagus and stomach. Once the tube is in place, the doctors can begin the treatment.

Compared to regular heartburn surgery, the endoscopic treatment won't cause any scars and offers faster recovery with lesser complications.

Before Making a Decision

If you are considering surgery as your heartburn treatment, you need to factor in the treatment costs and the pros and cons of each surgical treatment. Ask your doctor's opinion as to which surgery is most likely to produce the relief you seek. Of course, you also need to pick a surgical procedure you are comfortable with too.

If you are still confused about the surgery options, it is best to hold it off until you have the information and comfort you need to undergo the procedure. Examine your lifestyle and habits. Your heartburn may not be cured by medication because of your current lifestyle. Changing some of your habits could be the answer to curbing heartburn symptoms forever. It is preferable to make adjustments to your eating and exercise habits first, prior to undertaking a corrective surgical procedure.

Chapter 5: Lifestyle Changes To Cure

Heartburn

When it comes to heartburn, changes in your lifestyle can make a great difference. These modifications can help relieve symptoms and keep heartburn at bay with minimal help from medications.

Dietary Changes

Avoid food triggers

There are numerous food and drink items that aggravate heartburn. If you want to avoid the burning and painful sensation in your chest, you should avoid these food items:

1. Citrus fruits and tomatoes are very acidic and could cause instant heartburn especially when eaten on an empty stomach.

2. If you have severe heartburn, eating garlic and onions may trigger it. The same goes for spices. If you cannot avoid eating these food items, opt for the mildest choice or consume only a small portion.

3. Peppermint may freshen your breath but it could cause painful heartburn. This is because peppermint has properties that prompt the esophagus' sphincter muscle to relax thus allowing acid to flow back up. The same effect happens with chocolates so avoid them as well, if you can.

4. Food with high fat-content like meat, nuts, cheese and avocadoes are common heartburn triggers and must be eaten sparingly. Although not acidic, the fat in these food types slows down digestion and prompts the stomach to produce more acid.

Stop Overeating

Each time you eat a very large meal, your stomach stretches and puts a lot of pressure on your sphincter. This causes stomach acid production to increase to help digest the food faster. Unfortunately, too much acid can irritate your digestive system and causes acid reflux. Eat 6 small meals a day instead of 3 large ones. Smaller meals are digested faster so production of excess stomach acid is not necessary. This reduces the occurrence of heartburn.

Don't Eat then Sleep

Oftentimes, your heartburn acts up when you eat just before going to bed. Prevent that pain and discomfort by eating your meals at least 4 hours before going to bed at night. If you must eat late, make your meal small and wait 30 minutes before lying down.

Don't Rush

When eating, relax and chew your food properly. Count up to 20 before swallowing to ensure that your food is well chewed and then it can be more easily digested. Eating too fast or when stressed causes the stomach to produce more acid.

Limit Intake of Liquor, Carbonated and Caffeinated Drinks

Beer, hard liquor, coffee, energy drinks, tea, soda and similar drinks put a lot of pressure on your stomach that could cause acid reflex. Instead of consuming several cups of these drinks daily, limit yourself to one or two cups a day.

Chew Gum or Sour Balls

To prevent or ease the discomfort from heartburn, chew on a piece of gum or suck on sour balls and throat lozenges. This will help stimulate saliva production to lessen the presence of acid in the stomach.

Bedtime Habits

Sleep in a semi-upright position

Let stomach acid stay where it belongs with the help of gravity. Sleep with an extra pillow or a wedge pillow to elevate your upper body by 6 inches while sleeping. If you find this uncomfortable or if your posture is suffering, you can opt to place stacks of books under the head of the bed instead.

Sleep on your left side

Assuming this sleeping position helps reduce heartburn symptoms. When lying on your left side, your stomach creates a sharp angle that prevents acid from climbing back up to the esophagus.

Other Lifestyle Modifications

Quit Smoking - Nicotine found in cigarettes causes the lower esophageal sphincter to relax and that allows stomach acid to rise up.

Wear Looser Clothing - Constantly wearing tight clothes and belts puts a lot of pressure on your stomach especially during meals. The pressure causes stomach acid and contents to push through the sphincter muscles up to the esophagus.

Lose Weight - If you are overweight or obese, you naturally produce excessive amounts of stomach acid due to overeating or bingeing. The extra weight that you have also causes unnecessary pressure on your abdomen that pushes stomach acid up to the esophagus.

Keep Calm - Stress hastens the production of acid in the stomach. It doesn't just cause heartburn but could also lead to ulcers and other digestive problems. Avoid stressful situations at home or at work whenever you can and engage in relaxing activities like meditation, yoga, or any activity that you love to help you relax and de-stress.

Exercise - Keep heartburn at bay by engaging in activities that increase your heart rate. However, never exercise on a full stomach. It is best to wait about one hour or two before working out after eating.

Chapter 6: Home Remedies For Heartburn

Easing the aches of heartburn can be as easy as using items you probably already have in your kitchen. Home remedies are used by many sufferers because they are effective, all-natural, and safe. If you feel a burning sensation in your chest, your kitchen cupboard may have just what you need to ease the pain.

Baking Soda

As a natural antacid, baking soda can be used to relieve heartburn pain. Just dissolve about a teaspoon of baking soda in 8 ounces of water. Wait for the fizz to disappear before drinking it. Consume a baking soda drink once a day and only when you experience heartburn.

Herbal Tea

Like chamomile or fenugreek tea, there are many simple tea brews that you can concoct to ease heartburn pains including:

1. Ginger tea – In a cup of boiling water, add a teaspoon of freshly grated ginger root and let steep for 10-15 minutes before drinking.

2. Anise, fennel or caraway tea – Boil a cup of water and add two teaspoons of anise, fennel, or caraway seeds. Let steep for 10 minutes before straining the liquid. Drink while still warm.

3. Marshmallow root tea – The root of the marshmallow herb, scientific name Althea officinalis, contains properties that heal heartburn. Fill a jar (with lid) ¼ of the way with chopped marshmallow root. Fill the jar with lukewarm water and close the lid. After sitting overnight, the water should be thick, gooey, and yellowish. Strain and remove the roots before drinking. This cold drink stores for 3 days in the refrigerator.

Vegetable Juices

Juices extracted from raw celery, cabbage, and potato make great remedies for heartburn. These alkaline juices soothe the burning sensation in your chest immediately.

Aloe Vera Juice

Aloe vera is very popular for soothing an acidic stomach and an irritated esophagus. To begin making aloe vera juice, remove the skin of the aloe vera stem and peel of the initial yellow layer. Once the clear aloe vera gel is exposed, scoop all of it out and place it in a blender. Blend 2 teaspoons of gel with 8 ounces of water until smooth. Pour the drink in a glass and consume immediately.

Your miracle doctor, see http://engedi.info/AloeVera

Slippery Elm Tea

33

Drinking two to three cups of slippery elm daily helps thicken the mucous lining in your stomach as protection from acid. Just add one teaspoon of slippery elm powder to 8 ounces of water and drink.

Deglycyrrhizinated Licorice (DGL)

A type of herb licorice that's free of glycyrrhizin-related side effects, DGL helps ease heartburn by healing the stomach. It is available in capsules or chewable tablets. Doctors recommend taking one DGL capsule or tablet before meals.

Turmeric

A delicious spice, turmeric aids in digestion thus preventing the build-up of acid. If you dislike the taste of turmeric, you can buy turmeric capsules in different health stores.

Raw Almonds

Snacking on almonds eases heartburn symptoms since it produces alkaline that balances the pH level in the stomach.

Chapter 7: Cooking To Avoid Heartburn

When it comes to heartburn relief, prevention is key. If you find yourself suffering from that familiar and unwelcome burning sensation in your chest after every meal, you must take action to prevent it from happening again. Modify the way you prepare your food as well as the ingredients that you use. Doing so, you'll feel good, instead of pained, when your meal is over.

Keep these tips in mind:

1. Heartburn is aggravated by eating fatty meat. If you can't refrain from eating meat, always opt for leaner cuts of red meat such as tenderloin, chuck, sirloin or round. Chicken, turkey, and duck, although healthier than beef, pork or lamb, also contain fat. Choose white meat rather than dark. When preparing the meat, slice off any visible fat and discard the skin.

2. Some spices and flavorings can irritate the stomach and cause heartburn symptoms to appear. Steer clear of any hot spices such as chili powder, Tabasco sauce, and black or crushed pepper. Eliminate the use of raw onions and garlic and opt for small amounts of dried or dehydrated versions instead. To add flavor to your food, use tarragon, dill, basil, parsley, thyme, and cinnamon instead.

3. Tomatoes, citrus fruits, and vinegar can make heartburn worse so avoid it completely. Look for ingredient alternatives that you can use instead.

4. Consuming dairy products may be great for your bones but it could cause your heartburn to worsen. High in fat, dairy products stay in the stomach longer and cause a rapid production of stomach acid. To prevent a heartburn attack, choose low-fat or non-fat cheeses, yogurts, and sour creams instead. When cooking with cream or butter, use a reduced-fat cream or butter substitute.

5. For someone who is suffering from heartburn, you must be careful about how you cook your food. Eliminate the use of cooking oil and steer clear from your usual deep fry, pan-fry or sauté cooking methods. Prepare your food by steaming, grilling, roasting or broiling to avoid unnecessary fat without compromising flavor. Use more natural broths and juices rather than fats and oils.

6. Because heartburn always strikes after a meal, you should strictly practice portion control. Eating smaller portions may be hard but you'll get used to it in a few weeks. You'll even lose weight too!

7. Tip: Use a smaller plate to trick your mind and eye. A small plate full of food is definitely better than a large, but practically empty, one.

8. A portion-controlled meal means you'll still have room for dessert. Just skip chocolate and peppermint-flavored desserts altogether to

avoid triggering heartburn. Prepare luscious desserts made with vanilla, reduced-fat peanut butter, selected fruits and other low-fat ingredients.

As you are cooking delicious meals to avoid heartburn, always stock your pantry and fridge with the right ingredients. You should always buy more broths, high-fiber food items, and non-fat (or low fat) dairy products instead of the usual tomato-based sauces, oils, and refined grains. Practice the "out of sight, out of mind" method too. If you don't purchase and store chocolate, soda, frozen fried food, orange juice, and the likes, you won't think about eating them. When you do crave them, you'll be forced instead to cook a heartburn trigger-free meal because you won't have any of these food items in your home. A winning situation, don't you think?

Chapter 8: Delicious Recipes That Prevent

Heartburn

Whipping up delicious meals can be really frustrating if you have heartburn. Because of your limited ingredient choices, you tend to think you won't be able to indulge in delicious food anymore. But don't fret. There are numerous meals that you can easily make at home. These meals are not only delicious but help ease heartburn symptoms as well. Here are the recipes:

Breakfast

Walnut-Apricot Breakfast Bars

Serves: 16

Ingredients:

½ cup chopped walnuts, 2 cups dried apricots, 3 cups rolled oats, 3 cups puffed grain cereal (unsweetened), ¼ cup all-purpose flour, 12 ounce silken tofu (drained), 1 large egg, ½ cup canola oil, ½ teaspoon salt, 1 tablespoon vanilla extract, and 1 cup honey

Procedure: Preheat oven to 350 degree Fahrenheit. Using a cooking spray, lightly coat a jelly-roll pan.

Spread the walnuts and oats in a baking pan and bake for 8 to 10 minutes or until golden brown. Place in a large bowl and mix with the apricots, puffed cereal, salt and flour. Set aside.

Blend egg, tofu, oil, vanilla and honey until smooth. Pour in the oat mixture and mix thoroughly. Spread the combination in the prepared pan and bake for 35 to 40 minutes or until firm. Let cool in a wire rack before cutting into bars.

Lunch

Barley and Cream of Mushroom Soup

Serves: 4

Ingredients: 4 ½ cups reduced-sodium chicken broth, ½ cup pearl barley, 2 cups boiling water, 2 teaspoons butter substitute, 8 cups sliced white mushroom, 1 ounce porcini mushrooms (dried), 1 tablespoon extra virgin olive oil, 1 cup minced shallots, 2 celery stalks (finely chopped), ¼ cup fresh chives (minced), 1 tablespoon fresh sage (minced), 2 tablespoons all-purpose flour, ½ cup reduced-fat sour cream, 1 cup dry sherry, ½ teaspoon ground pepper, and ½ teaspoon salt

Procedure:

In a saucepan, boil barley in 1 ½ cups of broth in high heat. Cover pan, reduce heat and let simmer for 35 minutes.

Meanwhile, soak porcinis in boiling water until softened. Place soft mushrooms on paper towels. Once the mushrooms are dry, chop finely and set aside.

Heat oil and butter in a Dutch oven over medium-high heat and add the shallots. Next, stir in the white mushrooms until brown. Add the celery, sage, porcinis, salt and pepper. After 3 minutes, sprinkle the flour and combine. Stir in the sherry until somewhat evaporated.

Add the soaking liquid and remaining broth before turning heat to high. Once the soup has boiled, reduce heat and simmer for 20 minutes. Stir occasionally until thick. Add the barley until heated and stir in sour cream. Garnish with chives and serve immediately.

Dinner

Crispy Cod

Serves: 4

Ingredients:

4 skinless cod fillets, 24 Ritz crackers, 1 tablespoon butter, 3 tablespoons mayonnaise, 2 tablespoons curly parsley

(finely chopped), 2 garlic cloves (finely chopped), salt and pepper (to taste)

Procedure:

Position over rack in the middle of the oven and preheat to 450 degrees. Lightly grease baking sheet with butter and set aside.

In a medium-sized bowl, grind crackers into crumbs and add half of the parsley. Mix mayonnaise, remaining parsley and garlic in another bowl. Pat the cod fish dry with a paper towel before seasoning with salt and pepper. Position the fish on the buttered pan. Brush the sides and top of the fish with the mayo mixture before sprinkling the cracker crumbs on top.

Bake the cod until crispy and light brown. Serve immediately.

*If lemon isn't a heartburn trigger for you, you can squeeze a few drops on the fish before eating.

Snacks

Creamy Hummus Dip

Ingredients: 1 19-ounce can chickpeas (drained and washed), 2 tablespoons olive oil, 1 cup chicken stock, ½ teaspoon salt and ¼ teaspoon sesame oil

Procedure:

Put all the ingredients in a blender and process until creamy. Serve the dip cold with corn chips, flat bread or toast points.

Honeydew and Gala Apple Smoothie

Ingredients: 1 gala apple (peeled, cored and cut into pieces), 2 cups honeydew melon (peeled, seeded and cut into pieces), 4 tablespoons fresh aloe vera gel, 1 ½ cup ice, ¼ teaspoon salt and 1/16 teaspoon lime zest

Procedure:

Combine all the ingredients in the blender. Start blending on pulse before switching to medium and then high. Continue until mixture is smooth and creamy.

Banana Cupcakes with Cream Cheese

Makes: 12

Ingredients:

For cupcake- ½ cup mashed bananas (ripe), 1 cup flour, 4 egg whites, ¼ cup fat-free sour cream, ¼ teaspoon salt, ½ teaspoon baking soda, ¾ cup granulated sugar, ½ teaspoon ground cinnamon, and 1 teaspoon vanilla extract

For frosting - 8 ounces fat-free cream cheese (softened), 1 ½ cups powdered sugar, and 1 teaspoon vanilla extract

Procedure:

Preheat oven to 350 degrees Fahrenheit. Lightly spray a 12-cup muffin pan with low-fat, non-stick cooking spray. Stir flour, salt, cinnamon and baking soda in a bowl and set side.

In another bowl, cream butter and sugar together. Add the mashed bananas and vanilla. Whisk in egg whites and mix thoroughly. Stir in the sour cream and half of the flour mixture. Once blended, add the remaining flour mixture. Stir well.

Using a spoon, scoop just the right amount of butter into the greased muffin cups. Bake for 30-40 minutes or until done.

To make the frosting, combine all ingredients together and whisk until creamy.

Cool the cooked cupcakes for 15-20 minutes before removing them from the pan. Let cool for another hour before frosting.

Quick n' Easy Honey Banana Sorbet

Ingredients:

3 large bananas (peeled), 1/8 teaspoon ground cardamom, 1 tablespoon grated ginger root, 2 tablespoon honey, ¼ teaspoon salt and 3 cups ice

Procedure:

Place all ingredients, except the ice, in the blender and mix on high until creamy. Add the ice and blend well. Consume immediately.

Chapter 9: A Brief Introduction To Heartburn,

Its Causes And Symptoms

Do you suffer from a burning sensation in the middle of your chest after having your food? Then you may be suffering from an intestinal disease called heartburn scientifically known as GERD (Gastroesophageal reflux disease). Heartburn is a biological condition where the acid presenting in your stomach goes to the oesophagus, disrupting its normal functioning and giving you burning sensation. You would know that our stomach contains many acids to digest the food that we take like bile and several other digestive enzymes such as pepsin. Now, when these acids directly come into the contact with your oesophagus, it causes a burning sensation and agitation. The main function of our oesophagus is to send the food into the stomach, and the muscles of the oesophagus are very gentle so that the food you eat slips easily through to the stomach. There is a special one way valve that stops the acid going into the oesophagus, but due to some disruption; this doorway is unable to stop the acid going into your

48

oesophagus. This causes heartburns inside your stomach. The one way valve of the oesophagus is generally known as "Oesophageal sphincter" (LES), located at the bottom of the oesophagus. When the LES relaxes is weak or loose, and then the content of the stomach flows back into the oesophagus.

Your heartburn can become more severe in following cases: --

The LES's muscular tone.

Increase in the type and quantity of liquid that refluxes from your stomach.

Loss in the natural ability of your oesophagus muscle to cleanse its bottom.

The natural immune system of our body tries to minimize the damage to our oesophagus from acids by sending saliva. Saliva that contains water, mucus, enzymes, and electrolytes neutralizes that effect of acids and protects your oesophagus from any kind of damage and malfunctioning. But it has also some limitations since gravity pushes the liquid back into the stomach during the daytime when we are in upright position most of the time. Moreover, the problem still persists during the night since our body produces less saliva at night. Thus, the acids stay longer in the oesophagus increasing the damage and injury to the lining of the oesophagus.

Some Common Causes of Heartburn

After studying various patients of heartburn for a long period of time, the doctors have found that there seems to be a clear genetic tendency to develop heartburn, such as having a weak LES or hiatal hernia. Hiatal hernia is a biological condition where an oversized opening in the diaphragm occurs that makes it easier for the stomach, making it more prone to heartburn in the later stages. However, many hiatal hernia sufferers show no signs of reflux in many cases. So, doctors say that the real reasons of heartburn lie more in choice of lifestyle. Some medications and drugs that dilate the blood vessels such as calcium channel blockers may reduce the muscle tone of the LES, thereby making it more prone to heartburns. Smoking, drinking, and eating certain kind of processed foods are also some of the common reasons of heartburn since they can weaken and relax the LES. Heartburn is the outcome of unusual lifestyle that can contain eating processed and high fatty foods, not exercising, high amount of stress, and not taking proper sleep. Heartburn is most common after eating a large meal. A belly full of too much food can stretch your stomach, causing you to feel stuffed. This stretching or distention puts a lot of pressure on the LES, so juices from your last meal may come back to give you heartburns. Some fatty and processed foods can make your stomach more acidic, thereby increasing the candid growth, intoxicating the blood and the organs of elimination. This causes digestive problems and lead your body to fermentation that remains in your intestine for a long period of time and up to your oesophagus.

Pressure on your abdomen due to pregnancy, tight fitting attires, or obesity can also make you suffer from heartburns because the content of your stomach may flow back into the oesophagus due to excess pressure.

Heartburn is a complex medical condition triggered by one or more than one factors. This is the reason why it is not easy to control in many patients who are suffering from stress, obesity, or any other condition that is not easy to control. Doctors still find it difficult to control this chronic condition through the use of conventional drugs and medications. However, the natural and holistic approach to cure this condition is now considered to be the best way that tackles the problem from the root and restores the inner environment back into balance. In this book, we will learn how to control heartburn through natural means.

Chapter 10: Change In Diet And Dietary

Optimization To Cure Heartburn

1. Lowering Fat and Cholesterol

The higher amount of cholesterol and fat is not good for your health by any reason and it is one of the main triggers of heartburns. The first step towards lowering your fat would be to lose weight. Carrying high amount of fat is the main reason of heartburn since it puts a lot of pressure on the muscles of your stomach, thereby throwing acids into your oesophagus. Reducing your weight to around 5-10% can really lower your cholesterol levels. Just take an honest look at your eating habits and your routine calorie intake. It was found in many cases that if a person feels a lot of stress, then he pushes him to binge eating habits to get rid of that stress instead of finding a better cure. If you have the same condition and you think that you are binge eating, then try to give up your bingeing habit by applying a proper meal plan.

Living without food for a long period of time to lose weight is not a good approach according to many dieticians. Whenever you do dieting, next time the prospects of consuming more food increases by 50-80%, that implies you will feed the double sum of food next time. If you want to give up binge eating, you must understand the metabolic process of feeding and digestion in your torso. Our body's metabolic rate plays an important character to interpret the several processes of feeding and digestion. It is the pace at which your body processes food and converts it into fuel. If you forcefully restrict your food intake and then bust, and so it brings havoc to your metabolism. Repeatedly decreasing the quantity of nutrient intake can put your body in conversation mode and slow down your metabolism and your body won't function properly in this shell.

When planning your meal plan, think along the creases of your breakfast, lunch, and finally dinner. Add at least 2 snacks and something light before you get to bed. The basic motivation behind employing a meal plan is to replace the pattern of alternating between bingeing and dieting with a practice of steady eating. This gets a worrying process

for you and you can easily look after yourself
by watching your meal program.

A simple example of a meal plan: --

Time	Meal
8:30 AM	Breakfast
11:00 AM	Snack
01:00 PM	Lunch

04:00 PM	Snack
07:00 PM	Dinner
	Bedtime

The foods listed above in the meal plan are just a rough idea of your meal plan. Although, you are free to add or remove any food materials in this meal plan according to your choice or your body condition after reading this whole book.

Now, when you have devised a meal plan for yourself, the next step to cure your heartburn is your choice for healthy and nutritious food free from fat and cholesterol. One of the main reasons of increase in your cholesterol level is your choice of bad fat. You can use natural fats to lose cholesterol like olive, canola, and peanut oil. These fats contain natural Omega-

3 fatty acids that are beneficial for your heart and reduce the signs of ageing by reducing the amount of free radicals in your body. Avoid any kind of saturated fats found in red meat and dairy products.

Another harmful fat known as trans fat may be the reason of your obesity. Some of the commonly known trans fats are found in fried food products such as cookies, crackers, and snack cakes. Although, you can take some snacks made by baking and not frying as provided in your meal plan, but you must avoid any kind of fried food products containing trans fats.

Now, once you give up fats you also have to limit the amount of cholesterol you take through some foods. Aim for taking no more than 300mg of cholesterol a day; less than 200mg if you are suffering from heart disease or diabetes. Some of the sources of cholesterol are red meat, egg yolks, and dairy products, so stop consuming them. Omega-3 fatty acids found in some fishes like salmon, tuna, and mackerel are beneficial to reduce the amount of bad cholesterol in your body; that you have gained after eating junk and processed food. Almonds and walnuts are also a good source of Omega-3 fatty acids.

2. Increasing Fibre Intake

Taking a large amount of fibre from your food is the next step toward curing your heartburn. Fibre is also good for maintaining your digestive system by reducing bloating and constipation. Eating enough fibre from your food can feel you fuller for a whole day, so that you would not force yourself to eat unhealthy fast food. If you are an adult, then taking 30g of fibre from your food would be enough to keep your digestive system in pace. Now, there are mainly two kinds of fibre called soluble fibre and insoluble fibre. Soluble fibres are generally found in fruits, oats, and beans that can be easily digested in your stomach and intestines; forming a gel like substance when exposed to water. Soluble fibres are a must for you if you are obese and have digestive problems since they move waste products lurking inside your stomach for a long period of time through your digestive tract and they also help to lower your cholesterol level.

Insoluble fibres are generally found in wheat bran, grain, and cereals. They are insoluble in water and moves undigested through the intestinal tract. Insoluble fibres are beneficial because they can drain away insoluble impurities of your stomach and cleans it.

Fibres are good for curing heartburns because it can strengthen the muscles of your stomach and LES by providing it some exercising through movements and digestion. Your natural condition of opening the valve of your stomach can be retained by taking some soluble and insoluble fibres, so that the acids won't throw back to your oesophagus.

3. Reducing Spice Content in Your Food

You would have realized that taking a large chunk of spicy burger has increased your burning sensation. Spicy foods are one of the main reasons of heartburn because they imbalance the amount of digestive enzymes in your stomach, thereby pushing the acids into your oesophagus. You must avoid taking spicy food before sleeping because it can put many negative effects to your digestive system and your stomach's natural functioning. Spicy food can increase the body temperature and also blood pressure and that's why they may be the reason of your stress. So, you must reduce the amount of spicy food intake for naturally curing your heartburn.

Following are some tips to reduce the intake of spice in your food: --

You must avoid taking spice in your food to reduce the temperature of your body. If you are a soup lover then you can add broth or stock to tone down its heat.

Some good amount of yogurt of almond milk is helpful for you to give up an addiction to spice since they are natural sweet inhibitors, but avoid taking excess amount of dairy products because they are also not good for your digestion.

Eat green leafy vegetables and fruits as much as you can to give up your urge to eat spicy foods.

Avoid eating red meat and processed foods because they contain a large amount of spices that are not good for your stomach.

4. Reducing Gas Forming Foods

If you have a severe problem of gas, then it's sure that you will suffer from heartburns in future. Gas exerts a lot of pressure on the stomach and thereby some acid may throw out to the oesophagus to control the pressure. Passing out gas is a natural condition and don't bother if you are having passing out gas often, the problem persists when the gas traps inside your stomach and causes pressure. Most people pass gas or belch 20 times a day. But you must understand the excess is not plausible in case of anything, so try to control the amount of gas in your stomach, especially when you are already suffering from heartburns. Your body can produce gas for many reasons like for example swallowing too much gas or change in your diet. Now, swallowing too much air is often found among the smokers and drinkers. Smokers take a long shot of their favourite cigarette and inhales lots of harmful gases and some parts of these gases go directly to the stomach. These harmful gases trapped inside the stomach and causes pressure. People who drink beer and other beverages having gas are also prone to gas problems because they intake a lot of gas that traps inside their stomach. So, if you are a chain smoker or a drinker, then give up as soon as possible to retain your health and get rid of heartburns.

Here is a list of some food products that are responsible for gas formation: --

Milk and dairy products

Starchy food products like potatoes and pasta, especially fried ones

Wheat and oat bran

Artificially sweetened foods like soda, hard candy, or gum

Onions, green peppers, and scallions

Corn, celery, artichokes, and carrots

Remember that some amount of gas is beneficial for your body and you don't have to totally avoid each and every food material that produces gas. There are some special foods that are particularly responsible for making gas in some people and the combination is often different among different groups of people. So it is important that you find out which food product is most responsible for gas production in your case. Once you figured out which food cause you to suffer from excessive gas, it's time to limit them in your diet. Some of the food containing fibre that we discussed in the earlier section of the book is also responsible for gas production. If you have recently increased the amount of fibre in your diet, then you would face some gas problems, but don't worry since your body needs a couple of days to get used to the extra fibre and learn how to break it down.

If your gas problem is becoming more severe and effecting your digestion, then you can try some of the following natural remedies for gas cure: --

Add ½ tsp of cinnamon powder with a cup of warm milk, and honey, stir them together and drink.

Add 2 tsp of apple cider vinegar to a glass of lukewarm water and drink.

Mix equal parts of ginger, cardamom, and fennel. Add 1 tsp of this mixture, a pinch of asafetide (hing) to a cup of water and drink before going to sleep and at morning.

Chapter 11: Cleansing And Detoxification

1. Consuming Lots of Cleansing Foods

Cleansing our body from the impurities that deposit deep at many parts of our body is the main step for curing our heartburn. We eat many kinds of food materials and some of them have impurities that are not easily removable. We also intake large amount of impurities through our nostrils. So, cleansing is the best way to get rid of many impurities presenting inside our body. One of the main parts of our digestive system is a colon, which is a 5-6 foot long muscular tube that absorbs fluids and some nutrients. Any harmful effect on our colon directly impacts our digestive system, and thereby causing heartburn in many cases. So, our main purpose of cleansing is to clean our colon from impurities. Now, there are a variety of foods that are helpful to cleanse our colon and keep it functioning properly.

Here are some of the foods that are helpful to cleanse your colon: --

Raw green vegetables: -- Raw green vegetables are a must in your diet if you are looking to cure heartburn. However, the most beneficial part of raw green vegetables is that they are helpful to cleanse your colon. Our digestive system works in a precise way i.e. the digestive enzymes of our digestive system amalgamate with the digestive enzymes of food to break it down thoroughly. But as we become older, the ability of our digestive system diminishes and so the quantity of digestive enzymes inside our stomach decreases. This is the main reason why heartburn is a common disease among older people. Cooking the food at a higher temperature destroys the natural digestive enzymes of our food and that's why raw green vegetables are mandatory when you want to cure your heartburn problem, because then you can retain the natural enzymes of food and digest the food properly while eating it raw.

Foods containing fibre: -- I have already mentioned the benefits of fibre rich food in the earlier section of this book. Now I am emphasizing again on fibre rich food because they are also beneficial for the cleansing of your colon. Both soluble and insoluble fibres add bulk that gently stretches and stimulates the intestinal lining ensures healthy rhythmic muscular contractions that are helpful to move the food through your digestive tract. This rhythmic movement is also beneficial to prevent constipation. So eat lots of fibre in your food to cleanse your colon.

Probiotic foods: -- Do you know what are probiotic foods? Probiotic foods are the foods that contain a reasonable amount of some of the natural and healthy bacteria that live in our colon. These bacteria accelerate our digestion process and keep our colon healthy. Some of the probiotic foods such as yogurt, kimchi, and miso many species of beneficial bacteria like Bifidus and Lactobacillus. There is also a group of foods called "Inulin" that are being used by these bacteria as a food source like beans, flaxseed, apples, onions, and asparagus.

2. Cleansing Your Liver

Cleansing our blood is as important as cleansing other parts of our body. But our liver needs special cleansing because it is one of the most crucial parts inside human body.

The main function of the liver is to filter the blood coming from our digestive tract before it passes through the rest of your body. The liver also produces some essential proteins, detoxify chemicals, and metabolize drugs. Before you go for the liver cleansing diet, get a thorough check up for your liver and consult your dietician and take some suggestions for how to start your diet program. If you have any kinds of allergies, then avoid taking the food that causes your allergies. Here are some of the tips before beginning a liver cleanse diet: --

Don't follow the diet if you are pregnant, nursing, have any kind of cancer, or you have any liver disease or hepatitis.

Drink 2 large glasses of water in empty stomach every morning after you wake up. Add some juice or fresh lemon if you want. It will be more beneficial if you take a green smoothie recipe having raw vegetables. (Use any recipe from our list)

Avoid grains having gluten, especially wheat.

If you are on a heavy dieting and don't want to take any kind of heavy protein diet, then you can use protein powder smoothie. (You can add a scoop of Whey protein or any other protein of your choice in our smoothie recipes)

The main purpose of your liver cleanse is to remove the impurities of your body. If you take traditional food from the market, you won't fulfil your main motivation, so I would suggest you to use organic food for your liver cleanse. Organic foods are a bit expensive, but you can use them during your liver cleanse program for maximum results.

Here are some common foods that are helpful for cleansing your liver: --

Garlic

Grapefruit

Beetroots and carrots

Green leafy vegetables

Avocados

Apples

Olive oil

The best way to consume the liver cleansing foods is to make smoothies. Smoothies are a combination of one or more liver cleansing food with natural sweeteners. All you have to do is to find the best combination of the above described foods that tastes best. Mix them and take them in the morning. One more thing that you must take 2 glasses of water every morning with empty stomach.

Chapter 12: Ayurvedic Method To Cure

Heartburn

Ayurveda is one of the ancient medication techniques that are still celebrated in many theatrical roles in the world like India. Ayurveda is believed to be more than 10,000 years old and it has many herbal medicines that can heal several diseases like heartburns, Arthritis, diabetes, stress, and worry. Today, Ayurveda has been recognised as an efficient variety of medications and adopted by many international medical institutions. Many life saving medicines had mentioned in Ayurveda like "Sanjeevani" that can bring back life in dead person. Although, Sanjeevani is not available today, however, there are many medications that could be good for our wellness. Heartburns can be easily cured by some conventional methods of Ayurveda and you don't need to be an expert to apply Ayurveda because most of the methods explained in Ayurveda are easy and you can do them at your home.

1. Best Weapon of Ayurveda to Cure Heartburn: Fasting

I am sure that you should know about fasting. Fasting is the complete abstinence of your food for a certain period of time to make your digestion strong and give your stomach sometime to cure naturally from the effects of harmful chemicals and pesticides that you consume through your food. One of the common reasons of heartburn is the accumulation of waste and poisonous matter in our body that results from our habit of overeating. The majority of people nowadays eat too much and do nothing to properly digest their food, which results in unusual reactions inside our stomach and imbalance of the acids and enzymes that are being used for digestion. But when we deprive our body from food for a certain period of time, the organs of our digestive system, lungs, and kidneys are provided an opportunity to expel and unhamper the overload of accumulated waste from our stomach. It also leads to regeneration of blood as well as repair and regeneration of the cells and tissues of our body.

Duration of Fasting

The duration of fasting depends upon your age, severity of your heartburn, the earlier history of any disease, and the type of drugs you are taking or have taken earlier. Choosing correct duration for your fasting is mandatory since long period of fasting may be hazardous if you are not used to it. If you know nothing about fasting, then I would suggest you to start with 1-3 days of fasting and don't just starve yourself from food. You can take juices and smoothies within fasting period. Even if you are acquaint to fasting, don't fast for more than a week.

Method of Fasting

There are many kinds of fasting explained in the book of Ayurveda but all of them are not in the scope of this book. The best way to fast for you to cure heartburn is juice fasting. Juice fasting is also beneficial for you since I have already explained about some cleansing foods, fibre foods, and foods that you take to reduce formation of gas in the form of juices or smoothies. Choose the best combination of the fruits and vegetables and take them during your fasting period. This should be the best way to cure immediately from your heartburn and I am sure that you should feel the changes within a few weeks or months.

Lots of energy may spend during your fasting period in the process of elimination of harmful and poisonous impurities from your body. So, I would suggest you to take physical and mental rest during your fasting period. It has been realized in many cases that if a person is not accustomed to fasting take fruit juices for a long period of time, then toxic wastes enter his blood stream that affects the normal bodily functions. In that case, you may feel dizziness and vomiting, then you must immediately discontinue the fast and take cooked vegetables having adequate amount of roughage such as spinach and beets, until your body function becomes normal.

You may take normal morning walks and do some simple meditation of yoga during your fasting period to stay curious and healthy. Don't take cold water baths and use lukewarm water for bathing. Fasting sometimes causes a state of sleeplessness that you can overcome with warm tub bath. You can also drink 1-2 glasses of hot water before going to bed in this case.

The success of fast depends mainly upon how it has broken, which is the most significant phase after your fasting. Some of the main rules of fasting are: not overeating, and eating the food slowly and chewing it properly. If your transition from juicing to solid food is carefully planned, then I am sure that you won't face any discomfort. Take the solid foods that I have explained earlier in the fibre foods, gas reducing foods, and cleansing foods section for best results.

2. Some Yoga Exercises to Strengthen Your Digestion

The main cause of heartburns is indigestion due to imbalance of acids and enzymes of our stomach. If we can strengthen our digestion system through some means, then we are sure that our heartburn will cure naturally without any medication. Ayurveda has explained many yoga exercises that are beneficial for your digestion. Here are few of them: --

Kunjal or Vaman Dhoti: -- Kunjal is the natural process of cleansing the interior of your stomach. Drink 4-6 glasses of lukewarm water mixed with a pinch of salt early in the morning with empty stomach. Then stand up, bend forward, and insert the index and middle fingers of your right hand into your mouth until they touch your uvulva. Now tickle your uvulva until you feel vomiting sensation. The saline matter will come out of your vomit bringing up the bile and toxic matter with it. Repeat the process until you are sure that all the water has been vomited out. You can do this exercise once a week or whenever you feel necessary. Persons suffering from hyperacidity can do this exercise without salt. It is also beneficial for your headache, nervous weakness, chronic cold, and asthma. Don't do this if you are suffering from any kind of heart disease, high blood pressure, or ulcers.

Shavasana or "the dead body pose": -- Shavasana is one of the easiest and beneficial yoga exercises to strengthen your digestion and thereby curing your heartburn. Lie flat on your rear, feet comfortably part, arms and hands extended about six inches from the torso, palms upwards and fingers half-closed. Gently close your eyes. Begin by consciously and gradually slowing down every part and each muscle of the body; feet, legs, calves, knees, thighs, stomach, hips, back, hands, weapons system, breast, shoulders, neck, head and expression. Relax yourself completely feeling as if your whole body is lifeless. Now concentrate your mind on breathing rhythmically as slowly and effortlessly as possible. This creates a state of complete relaxation. Remain motionless in this position, relinquishing all responsibilities and worries for 10 to 15 transactions. Discontinue the exercise when your legs grow numb.

Vajrasan (Pelvic pose exercise): -- Sit erect and stretch out your legs. Close your legs back, positioning the feet on the sides of the buns with the soles facing back and upwards. Rest your bottom on the level between your heels. The toes of both feet should touch. Straight off, put your hands on your knees and hold open the spine, neck and head straight. Vajrasana can be done even after meals. It improves the digestion and is beneficial in cases of dyspepsia, constipation, colitis, seminal weakness and stiffness of the legs. It strengthens the hips, thighs, knees, calves, ankles and toes.

Anuloma-viloma: -- Anuloma viloma is the most beneficial yoga for strengthening digestion. It is considered as a nadi shuddi pranayam (pulse purification exercise). Sit in a comfortable meditation position while keeping your head, neck, and spine erect. Now rest your left hand on your left knee. Close your right nostrils by pressing the tip of your right thumb against it. Now take a deep breath with your left nostril, while keeping your right nostril closed. Now repeat the same process while your left nostril closed. Repeat the entire process and inhale and exhale slowly without making any sound. This pranayma is best for curing your heartburns since it strengthen your oesophagus that is connected with your breathing nostrils.

All the exercise explained above are easy and you can do them at your home. However, you must consult your doctor if you are suffering from any kind of heart disease or breathing problems before attempting them at your home. You can also see the videos to know how to do these yoga exercises properly and easily. So follow the tips that I have shared with you in my book and live a heartburn free life. I am sure that you won't need any kind of medication and expensive surgeries if you follow the steps in this book precisely.

Chapter 13: Causes

A correlation of a solid condition to GERD

Indigestion is because of unfortunate conclusion of the lower esophageal sphincter, which is at the intersection between the stomach and the esophagus. Factors that can add to GERD:

Hiatal Hernia,

Which improves the probability of GERD due to mechanical and motility factors.

Corpulence

Expanding weight record is related with more serious GERD. In an enormous series of 2,000 patients with suggestive reflux disease, it has been shown that 13% of changes in esophageal corrosive openness is owing to changes in weight index.

Factors that have been connected with GERD, yet not convincingly:

Obstructive Rest Apnea

Gallstones, which can hinder the progression of bile into the duodenum, which can influence the capacity to kill gastric acid[medical reference needed]

By and large, 40% of GERD patients additionally had H. pylori infection. The destruction of H. pylori can prompt an expansion in corrosive secretion, prompting whether or not H. pylori-contaminated GERD patients are any not quite the same as non-tainted GERD patients. A twofold visually impaired study, revealed in 2004, found no clinically tremendous contrast between these two sorts of patients concerning the emotional or objective proportions of disease severity.

Endoscopic picture of peptic injury, or restricting of the throat close to the intersection with the stomach: This is an entanglement of persistent gastroesophageal reflux infection and can be a reason for dysphagia or trouble gulping.

The determination of GERD is generally made when average side effects are present. Reflux can be available in individuals without side effects and the finding requires the two side effects or confusions and reflux of stomach content.

Other causes are

are overweight or hefty

are pregnant

have diabetes

smoke

Chapter 14: Signs And Symptoms

The most well-known side effects of GERD in grown-ups are an acidic desire for the mouth, disgorging, and heartburn. Less normal side effects incorporate agony with gulping/sore throat, expanded salivation (otherwise called water reckless), nausea, chest torment, hacking, and globus sensation. The heartburn can prompt asthma assault side effects like windedness, hack, and wheezing in those with basic asthma.

GERD some of the time makes injury the throat. These wounds might incorporate at least one of the accompanying:

Reflux Esophagitis

Aggravation of esophageal epithelium which can cause ulcers close to the intersection of the stomach and esophagus.

Esophageal Injuries

The relentless restricting of the throat brought about by reflux-prompted irritation.

Barrett's Throat

Digestive metaplasia (changes of the epithelial cells from squamous to gastrointestinal columnar epithelium) of the distal esophagus.

Esophageal Adenocarcinoma

A type of cancer

GERD now and again causes injury of the larynx (LPR). Other complexities can incorporate yearning pneumonia.

GERD might be challenging to recognize in babies and kids since they can't depict what they are feeling and markers should be noticed. Side effects might shift from regular grown-up side effects. GERD in kids might cause continued spewing, easy throwing up, hacking, and other respiratory issues, for example, wheezing. Hopeless crying, declining food, sobbing for food and afterward pulling off the container or bosom just to sob for it once more, inability to put on sufficient weight, terrible breath, and burping are likewise normal. Youngsters might have one side effect or many; no single side effect is general in all kids with GERD.

Of the assessed 4 million children brought into the world in the US every year, up to 35% of them might experience issues with reflux in the initial not many months of their lives, known as 'spitting up'.[21] About 90% of babies will grow out of their reflux by their first birthday.

Your stomach corrosive upholds into your throat. Your throat is the strong cylinder that associates your throat and stomach. The most widely recognized side effect of heartburn is a consuming sensation in your chest, known as acid reflux. Different side effects might incorporate a sharp or spewed food taste toward the rear of your mouth.

Indigestion is otherwise called gastroesophageal reflux (GER). On the off chance that you experience it over two times every week, you might have gastroesophageal reflux disease (GERD). Notwithstanding successive indigestion, side effects of GERD incorporate trouble gulping, hacking or wheezing, and chest torment.

Side Effects Of Gerd Include:

terrible breath

harm to tooth finish because of overabundance corrosive

indigestion

feeling like stomach contents have returned up to the throat or mouth, or disgorging

chest torment

steady dry hack

asthma

inconvenience gulping.

Chapter 15: Management And Treatment

Treatment choices incorporate way of life changes, meds, and at times a medical procedure for the people who don't improve with the initial two measures. Way of life changes incorporate not resting for three hours subsequent to eating, resting on the left side, raising the cushion/bedhead level, getting more fit, staying away from food sources which bring about side effects, and halting smoking. Medications incorporate acid neutralizers, H2 receptor blockers, proton siphon inhibitors, and prokinetics.

Treatment for acid reflux might incorporate drugs and dietary changes. Medication incorporate stomach settling agents. Dietary changes might require staying away from food varieties that are high in fats, fiery, high in fake flavors, weighty diminishing NSAID use, weighty liquor utilization, and diminishing peppermint consumption. Lifestyle changes might help like decreasing weight.

Other normal descriptors for indigestion (other than consuming) are burping, disease, crushing, cutting, or a vibe of strain on the chest. The aggravation frequently ascends in the chest (straightforwardly behind the breastbone) and may transmit to the neck, throat, or point of the arm. Since the chest houses other significant organs other than the throat (counting the heart and lungs), it is essential to recollect that not all side effects connected with acid reflux are esophageal in nature.

The reason will change contingent upon one's family and clinical history, hereditary qualities, in the event that an individual is pregnant or lactating, and age. Accordingly, the finding will shift contingent upon the thought organ and the instigating disease process. Stir up will fluctuate contingent upon the clinical doubt of the supplier seeing the patient, yet for the most part incorporates endoscopy and a preliminary of stomach settling agents to evaluate for relief.[citation needed]

The medicines for GERD might incorporate food decisions, way of life changes, prescriptions, and potentially medical procedure. Starting treatment is habitually with a proton-siphon inhibitor, for example, omeprazole at times, an individual with GERD side effects can oversee them by assuming control non-prescription drugs. This is frequently more secure and more affordable than taking doctor prescribed drugs. Some rules prescribe attempting to treat side effects with a H2 bad guy prior to utilizing a proton-siphon inhibitor due to cost and wellbeing concerns.

Certain food sources might advance GERD, yet most dietary mediations have little effect. Some proof proposes that decreased sugar consumption and expanded fiber admission can help. Avoidance of explicit food varieties and not eating prior to resting are suggested for those having GERD symptoms.[39] Foods that might encourage GERD incorporate espresso, liquor, chocolate, greasy food sources, acidic food varieties, and hot foods.

Food sources That May Cause Heartburn

Food sources ordinarily known to be acid reflux triggers make the esophageal sphincter unwind and postpone the stomach related process, allowing food to sit in the stomach longer, says Gupta. The most terrible guilty parties? Food varieties that are high in fat, salt or flavor, for example,

Broiled food

Cheap food

Pizza

Potato chips and other handled snacks

Stew powder and pepper (white, dark, cayenne)

Greasy meats like bacon and hotdog

Cheddar

Different food sources that can cause a similar issue include:

Tomato-based sauces

Citrus natural products

Chocolate

Peppermint

Carbonated drinks

"Control is key since many individuals will most likely be unable to or need to totally take out these food sources," says Gupta. "Yet, attempt to try not to eat issue food sources late at night nearer to sleep time, so they're not sitting in your stomach and afterward coming up your throat when you set down around evening time. It's likewise smart to eat little regular feasts rather than greater, heavier feasts and keep away from late-night meals and sleep time snacks."

Food sources That Help Prevent Acid Reflux

There are a lot of things you can eat to assist with forestalling indigestion. Stock your kitchen with food varieties from these three classifications:

a bowl of banana oats

High-fiber food sources

Stringy food sources encourage you so you're more averse to gorge, which might add to acid reflux. Thus, load up on solid fiber from these food varieties:

Entire grains like oats, couscous and earthy colored rice.

Root vegetables like yams, carrots and beets.

Green vegetables like asparagus, broccoli and green beans.

a bowl of blended nuts

Soluble food varieties

Food sources fall some place along the pH scale (a sign of corrosive levels). Those that have a low pH are acidic and bound to cause reflux. Those with higher pH are basic and can assist with areas of strength for balancing corrosive. Antacid food sources include:

Bananas

Melons

Cauliflower

Fennel

Nuts

a bowl of cut watermelon

Watery food sources

Eating food sources that contain a great deal of water can weaken and debilitate stomach corrosive. Pick food sources, for example,

Celery

Cucumber

Lettuce

Watermelon

Stock based soups

Natural tea

Acid reflux Home Remedies

Individuals with indigestion generally go after stomach settling agents, non-prescription drugs that kill stomach corrosive. Be that as it may, eating specific food varieties may likewise offer help from side effects. Think about attempting the accompanying:

milk emptying from a pitcher into a glass

Milk

Does drain assist with indigestion? "Milk is many times remembered to alleviate indigestion," says Gupta. "However, you need to remember that milk comes in various assortments — entire milk with everything of fat, 2% fat, and skim or nonfat milk. The fat in milk can disturb heartburn. Yet, nonfat milk can go about as a transitory cushion between the stomach lining and acidic stomach contents and give quick help of indigestion side effects." Low-fat yogurt has similar mitigating characteristics alongside a sound portion of probiotics (great microorganisms that improve processing).

some ginger tea

Ginger

Ginger is one of the most mind-blowing stomach related helps in view of its restorative properties. It's antacid in nature and mitigating, which facilitates disturbance in the gastrointestinal system. Have a go at tasting ginger tea when you feel indigestion coming on.

Apple juice vinegar and apples

Apple juice vinegar

While there isn't sufficient examination to demonstrate that drinking apple juice vinegar works for heartburn, many individuals swear that it makes a difference. Nonetheless, you ought to never drink it at full focus since areas of strength for a can disturb the throat. All things being equal, put a limited quantity in warm water and drink it with feasts.

some lemon water with honey

Lemon water

Lemon juice is by and large thought to be exceptionally acidic, however a modest quantity of lemon juice blended in with warm water and honey has an alkalizing impact that kills stomach corrosive. Additionally, honey has regular cancer prevention agents, which safeguard the wellbeing of cells

Weight reduction might be compelling in lessening the seriousness and recurrence of symptoms. Elevating the top of the whole bed with blocks, or utilizing a wedge pad that lifts the singular's shoulders and head, may repress GERD while lying down. Although moderate activity might further develop side effects in individuals with GERD, enthusiastic activity might deteriorate them. Breathing activities might ease GERD symptoms.

Restraint from smoking or liquor doesn't appear to altogether alleviate symptoms.

Prescriptions

Drugs for corrosive related messes

The essential prescriptions utilized for GERD are proton-siphon inhibitors, H2 receptor blockers and acid neutralizers despite everything alginic acid. The utilization of corrosive concealment treatment is a typical reaction to GERD side effects and many individuals get a greater amount of this sort of treatment than their case merits. The abuse of corrosive concealment is an issue due to the secondary effects and costs.

Dietary problems, for example, anorexia and bulimia nervosa, may likewise add to certain instances of GERD. Individuals who prompt retching, or have before, can have an expanded gamble of acid reflux.

Incidental or gentle instances of heartburn can generally be forestalled by embracing a couple of way of life changes. For instance:

Try not to rests for three hours after a feast.

Eat more modest feasts all the more oftentimes over the course of the day.

Wear baggy apparel to keep away from tension on your midsection.

Lose overabundance weight.

Stop smoking.

Raise the top of your bed six to eight creeps by putting wooden blocks under your bedposts. Bed risers are one more choice for doing this.

A few sorts of food can cause indigestion and acid reflux. Give close consideration to how you feel in the wake of eating various food sources. Your triggers might include:

greasy or seared food sources

liquor

espresso

carbonated refreshments, like pop

chocolate

garlic

onions

citrus organic products

peppermint

spearmint

pureed tomatoes

Assuming that you experience indigestion or acid reflux in the wake of eating specific food varieties, do whatever it takes to keep away from them.

The following are 14 normal ways of decreasing your indigestion and acid reflux, all upheld by logical exploration.

1. Bite Gum

A couple of more seasoned examinations have shown that biting gum might assist with diminishing causticity in the throat. Gum that contains bicarbonate seems, by all accounts, to be particularly compelling, as it can assist with killing corrosive to forestall reflux. Biting gum can likewise increment spit creation, which might assist with getting the throat free from corrosive. In any case, more cutting-edge research is expected to decide if biting gum can assist with treating heartburn or let the side effects free from acid reflux. Biting gum builds the arrangement of spit and may assist with getting the throat free from stomach corrosive.

2. Rest on your left side

A few investigations have discovered that dozing on your right side might deteriorate reflux side effects around evening time. As a matter of fact, as per one survey, lying on your left side might diminish corrosive openness in the throat by up to 71%. Albeit the explanation isn't altogether clear, it very well may be made sense of by life systems. The throat enters the right half of the stomach. Accordingly, the lower esophageal sphincter sits over the degree of stomach corrosive when you rest on your left side. Then again, when you lie on your right side, stomach corrosive covers the lower esophageal sphincter, expanding the gamble of reflux. While resting on the left side all night may not generally be imaginable, it could assist with making you more agreeable as you nod off. On the off chance that you experience heartburn around evening time, take a stab at dozing on the left half of your body.

3. Lift The Top Of Your Bed

Certain individuals experience reflux side effects during the evening, which can influence rest quality and make it more challenging to nod off. Changing the place that you stay in bed by lifting the top of your bed could assist with lessening side effects of heartburn and further develop rest quality.

3. Hoist The Top Of Your Bed

Certain individuals experience reflux side effects during the evening, which can influence rest quality and make it more hard to nod off. Changing the place that you snooze by hoisting the top of your bed could assist with lessening side effects of indigestion and further develop rest quality. One survey of four examinations found that lifting the top of the bed diminished indigestion and further developed side effects like acid reflux and disgorging in individuals with GERD. Another review showed that individuals who utilized a wedge to hoist their chest area while resting experienced less indigestion contrasted and when they dozed level.

Lifting the top of your bed might decrease your reflux side effects around evening time.

4. Have Supper Prior

Medical services experts frequently encourage individuals with heartburn to try not to eat inside the 3 hours before they fall asleep. That is on the grounds that lying on a level plane after a dinner makes processing more troublesome, possibly deteriorating GERD side effects. As per one survey, eating a late-night dinner expanded corrosive openness while resting by 5%, contrasted and eating prior at night.

Another review incorporating 817 individuals with type 2 diabetes observed that having supper late around evening time was related with a higher gamble of indigestion. In any case, more examinations are required before strong ends can be made about the impact of late night dinners on GERD. It might likewise rely upon the person.

Observational investigations recommend that eating near sleep time might deteriorate heartburn side effects around evening time.

Be that as it may, the proof is uncertain, and more investigations are required.

5. Select Cooked Onions Rather Than Crude

Crude onions are a typical trigger for indigestion and indigestion. One more seasoned concentrate on in individuals with indigestion showed that eating a feast containing crude onion essentially expanded acid reflux, heartburn, and burping, contrasted and consuming an indistinguishable dinner that didn't contain onions. More regular burping could recommend that more gas is being delivered. This could be because of the great measures of fermentable fiber in onions. Crude onions are likewise more challenging to process and could aggravate the coating of the throat, causing deteriorated indigestion. Whatever the explanation, on the off chance that you think eating crude onion aggravates your side effects, you ought to keep away from it and pick cooked onions all things considered.

Certain individuals experience deteriorated indigestion and other reflux side effects in the wake of eating crude onions.

6. Eat More Modest, More Regular Feasts

There's a ring-like muscle known as the lower esophageal sphincter where the throat opens into the stomach. It goes about as a valve and regularly forestalls the acidic items in the stomach from going up into the throat. It regularly remains shut however may open when you swallow, burp, or regurgitation. In individuals with heartburn, this muscle is debilitated or broken. Indigestion can likewise happen when there's an excess of tension on the muscle, making corrosive just barely get through the opening. Obviously, most reflux side effects occur after a dinner. It additionally appears to be that eating only one to two enormous dinners each day might deteriorate reflux side effects.

Thusly, eating more modest, more continuous feasts over the course of the day might assist with diminishing side effects of indigestion.

Indigestion generally increments after feasts, and bigger dinners appear to aggravate it. Consequently, eating more modest, more successive dinners might be valuable.

7. Keep a moderate weight

The stomach is a muscle situated over your stomach. Ordinarily, the stomach normally fortifies the lower esophageal sphincter, which keeps extreme measures of stomach corrosive from spilling up into the throat. In any case, assuming you have abundance tummy fat, the strain in your midsection might turn out to be high to such an extent that the lower esophageal sphincter gets pushed vertical, away from the stomach's help.

This condition, known as hiatal hernia, is viewed as the main source of GERD.

Moreover, research shows that having overabundance stomach fat might be related with a higher gamble of heartburn and GERD. Hence, a few examinations recommend that losing no less than 10% of your body weight could essentially diminish side effects of GERD in individuals with the condition. Accomplishing and keeping a moderate body weight can assist with diminishing heartburn in the long haul.

Be that as it may, in the event that you're keen on this methodology, make a point to talk with a medical services proficient to evaluate whether it's ideal for you, and provided that this is true, how you can get thinner securely and reasonably.

Losing gut fat and keeping a moderate weight could free some from your side effects of GERD. Nonetheless, make a point to talk with a medical services proficient prior to endeavoring to get more fit to treat this condition.

8. Follow A Low Carb Diet

Developing proof recommends that low carb diets might ease indigestion side effects. As a matter of fact, a few scientists suspect that undigested carbs may cause bacterial excess and expanded tension inside the midsection, which could add to heartburn. Having an excessive number of undigested carbs in your stomach related framework frequently could not just objective at any point gas and swelling yet additionally burping.

In any case, while certain examinations propose that low carb diets could further develop reflux side effects, more exploration is required.

Some exploration recommends that poor carb assimilation and bacterial excess in the small digestive tract might bring about heartburn. Low carb diets might be a powerful treatment, yet further investigations are required.

9. Limit your liquor admission

Drinking liquor might expand the seriousness of indigestion and acid reflux.

As a matter of fact, a few examinations have demonstrated the way that higher liquor admission could be connected to expanded side effects of indigestion. Liquor exasperates side effects by expanding stomach corrosive, loosening up the lower esophageal sphincter, and weakening the capacity of the throat to get out corrosive. Albeit new examination is required, a few more established investigations likewise show that drinking wine or lager increments reflux side effects, particularly contrasted and drinking plain water.

Inordinate liquor admission can demolish heartburn side effects. On the off chance that you experience acid reflux, restricting your liquor admission could assist with facilitating a portion of your inconvenience.

10. Try Not To Drink A Lot Of Espresso

Investigations have discovered that espresso briefly loosens up the lower esophageal sphincter, expanding the gamble of indigestion. Some proof likewise highlights caffeine as a potential reason. Comparably to espresso, caffeine loosens up the lower esophageal sphincter, which could cause reflux. By and by, albeit a few investigations recommend that espresso and caffeine might deteriorate heartburn for certain individuals, the proof isn't totally decisive.

For instance, one investigation of observational examinations tracked down no huge impacts of espresso consumption on oneself announced side effects of GERD. However, when specialists explored the indications of heartburn with a little camera, they found espresso utilization was connected to more prominent corrosive harm in the throat.

In this way, whether espresso admission demolishes heartburn might rely upon the person. Assuming you find espresso gives you indigestion, it's ideal to keep away from it or breaking point your admission basically.

Proof proposes that espresso might aggravate indigestion. Assuming that you feel like espresso deteriorates your side effects, think about restricting your admission.

11. Limit your admission of carbonated drinks

Medical services experts some of the time encourage individuals with GERD to restrict their admission of carbonated refreshments.

This is on the grounds that reviews have seen that standard utilization of carbonated or bubbly refreshments, including sodas, club pop, and seltzer, could be connected to a higher gamble of reflux. One investigation discovered that carbonated soda pops, specifically, demolished specific indigestion side effects, including acid reflux, totality, and burping.

The primary explanation is that the carbon dioxide gas (the air pockets) in carbonated drinks makes individuals burp more regularly — an impact that can build how much corrosive getting away into the throat

Drinking carbonated refreshments briefly builds the recurrence of burping, which might advance indigestion. Assuming they demolish your side effects, have a go at drinking less or keeping away from them out and out.

12. Try not to drink a lot of citrus juice

Many sorts of citrus juice, including squeezed orange and grapefruit juice, are viewed as normal triggers for indigestion. These fixings are exceptionally acidic and contain intensifies like ascorbic corrosive, which could cause heartburn on the off chance that you consume them in enormous sums. As well as being acidic, certain mixtures found in citrus juice could aggravate the coating of the throat. While citrus squeeze most likely doesn't cause indigestion straightforwardly, it could exacerbate your acid reflux briefly.

Certain individuals with heartburn report that drinking citrus juice aggravates their side effects. Certain mixtures in citrus juice, notwithstanding acids, can likewise disturb the covering of the throat.

13. Keep Away From Mint, If Necessary

Peppermint and spearmint are normal fixings used to make natural tea and add flavor to food sources, treats, biting gum, mouthwash, and toothpaste. Nonetheless, they additionally contain specific mixtures that could set off acid reflux in certain individuals. For example, a few investigations demonstrate that peppermint oil could diminish lower esophageal sphincter pressure, which might cause indigestion. One more review demonstrated the way that menthol, a compound saw as in mint, could deteriorate reflux in individuals with GERD.

Furthermore, one more seasoned concentrate on in individuals with GERD showed that spearmint didn't influence the lower esophageal sphincter. By the by, it found that high portions of spearmint could deteriorate heartburn side effects by disturbing within the throat. Consequently, it's ideal to keep away from mint assuming you feel that it exacerbates your acid reflux.

A couple of studies show that mint and a portion of the mixtures it contains may bother indigestion and other reflux side effects, yet the proof is restricted.

14. Limit High Fat Food Sources

Seared food varieties and a few other greasy food sources may likewise be a trigger for GERD. Some exploration shows they might prompt indigestion. Models incorporate

broiled food varieties

potato chips

pizza

bacon

wiener

High fat food sources like these may add to indigestion by causing bile salts to be delivered into your intestinal system, which might aggravate your throat.

They likewise seem to animate the arrival of cholecystokinin (CCK), a chemical in your circulation system that might loosen up the lower esophageal sphincter, permitting stomach contents once more into the throat.

One review saw what happened when individuals with GERD ate high fat food varieties. The greater part of members who had revealed food triggers said they encountered GERD side effects in the wake of eating high fat, seared food sources.

In addition, when these individuals dispensed with setting off food sources from their eating regimen, the extent of the people who experienced acid reflux diminished from 93% to 44%.

More examination is expected to reveal how high fat food varieties could set off GERD side effects, including indigestion, as well as what sorts of fats could make the most grounded impacts.

It's vital to take note of that fats are a fundamental piece of a sound eating routine. As opposed to keeping away from fats, mean to eat them with some restraint from sound sources, like omega-3 unsaturated fats from greasy fish and monounsaturated fats from olive oil or avocados.

Food sources that are high in fat might set off GERD side effects, including acid reflux, in certain individuals. Be that as it may, more exploration is required.

Chapter 16: Heartburn, Gerd, Indigestion

And Acid Reflux

The terms indigestion, heartburn, and GERD are frequently utilized conversely. They really have altogether different implications.

Heartburn is a typical ailment that can go in seriousness from gentle to serious. Gastroesophageal reflux disease (GERD) is the persistent, more serious type of indigestion. Indigestion is a side effect of heartburn and GERD.

The expression "indigestion" is misdirecting. The heart doesn't really have anything to do with the aggravation.

Acid reflux happens in your stomach related framework. In particular, in your throat. Acid reflux includes gentle to serious agony in the chest. It's occasionally confused with coronary episode torment.

The covering of your throat is more fragile than the coating of your stomach. Thus, the corrosive in your throat creates a consuming uproar in your chest. The aggravation can feel sharp, consuming, or like a fixing sensation. Certain individuals might portray indigestion as copying that climbs around the neck and throat or as distress that feels like it's situated behind the breastbone.

Indigestion typically happens subsequent to eating. Twisting around or resting can exacerbate it.

Indigestion is very normal. It is assessed that in excess of 60 million Americans experience indigestion something like one time per month. You might have the option to deal with your acid reflux by:

getting more fit

halting smoking

eating less greasy food varieties

staying away from fiery or acidic food varieties

Gentle, rare acid reflux can likewise be treated with drugs like stomach settling agents. In the event that you take acid neutralizers in excess of a few times each week a specialist ought to assess you. Your indigestion might be a side effect of a more serious issue like heartburn or GERD.

A round muscle called the lower esophageal sphincter (LES) joins your throat and stomach. This muscle is accountable for fixing your throat after food passes to the stomach. On the off chance that this muscle is frail or doesn't fix as expected, the corrosive from your stomach can go in reverse into your throat. This is known as indigestion.

Indigestion can cause acid reflux and different side effects that include:

hack

sore throat

harsh desire for the rear of the throat

118

acrid desire for the mouth

consuming and pressure that can stretch out up the breastbone

A great many people can encounter indigestion and heartburn irregularly connected with something they ate or propensities like resting following eating. Notwithstanding, GERD is an ongoing condition where specialists begin to inspect dependable propensities and portions of an individual's life systems that could cause GERD. Instances of the reasons for GERD include:

being overweight or fat, which comes down on the stomach

hiatal hernia, which diminishes tension in the LES

smoking

polishing off liquor

pregnancy

taking prescriptions known to debilitate the LES, for example, allergy meds, calcium channel blockers, torment alleviating medications, narcotics, and antidepressants

Side effects of GERD might upset your regular routine. Luckily, they can generally be controlled with treatment. Choices include:

diet adjustment

weight reduction

smoking end

liquor end

Indigestion happens when the items in your stomach back up into your throat. This happens when your lower esophageal sphincter (LES) unwinds and permits stomach corrosive to rise.

A few food-related variables might add to indigestion, for example, the place of your body in the wake of eating

how much food you eat during a solitary dinner

the sort of food sources you eat

You can deal with every one of these variables by altering how and what you eat. Basically moving your body position to an upstanding stance after a dinner and eating more modest parts might assist with forestalling reflux.

Knowing which food sources to stay away from can be a smidgen really confounding. There's still some discussion in the clinical local area over which food varieties really cause reflux side effects.

In spite of this absence of agreement, numerous analysts concur that it's ideal to keep away from specific kinds of food varieties and refreshments to forestall heartburn and different side effects of indigestion.

High fat dinners and seared food varieties

Greasy food sources for the most part lower strain on your LES and defer stomach purging. This might build your gamble for reflux side effects, as per the National Institute of Diabetes and Digestive and Kidney Diseases.

To assist with forestalling reflux, you can take a stab at diminishing your all out fat admission.

Here are a few high fat food sources you might need to keep away from:

french fries

broiled onion rings

potato chips

margarine

entire milk

cheddar

frozen yogurt

high fat harsh cream

high fat velvety serving of mixed greens dressings

velvety sauces and plunges

high fat cuts of red meat, like marbled sirloin or prime rib

Zesty food varieties

Review have proposed that zesty food sources can cause stomach torment and consuming side effects on the off chance that you have a practical gastrointestinal problem.

Capsaicin, the synthetic compound that makes food taste zesty, can bother portions of the throat, which can bring about heartburn.

As a matter of fact, a 2017 Korean study discovered that hot, hot stews prompted GERD side effects in the greater part of surveyed cases.

However a 2010 study recommended that individuals who routinely eat zesty food experience less GERD side effects from these feasts, there has been little exploration since to help this case.

• It's by and large most secure to stay away from hot food varieties assuming that you consistently experience indigestion.

Foods grown from the ground

Foods grown from the ground are a significant piece of your eating regimen. Nonetheless, particular sorts could aggravate your GERD. The accompanying products of the soil generally lead to reflux:

pineapple

citrus natural products, like oranges, grapefruit, lemons, and limes

tomatoes (and tomato-based food varieties)

garlic and onions

If all else fails, examine your resilience level with a specialist. On the off chance that you approach, a dietitian might help you in making an example of eating that can assist with dealing with your condition.

Refreshments

A few normal beverages may likewise set off side effects in individuals with GERD. These include:

liquor

espresso and tea

carbonated drinks

citrus and tomato juices

Regardless of caffeine, espresso could advance reflux side effects. Nonetheless, certain individuals with GERD endure espresso well.

Focus on your singular side effects and consume just refreshments that you endure well.

A few food-related variables might add to heartburn, for example,

the place of your body in the wake of eating

how much food you eat during a solitary dinner

the sort of food sources you eat

You can deal with every one of these variables by changing how and what you eat. Essentially moving your body position to an upstanding stance after a feast and eating more modest segments might assist with forestalling reflux.

Knowing which food varieties to stay away from can be somewhat really confounding. There's still some debate in the clinical local area over which food sources really cause reflux side effects.

In spite of this absence of agreement, numerous specialists concur that it's ideal to stay away from specific sorts of food varieties and drinks to forestall heartburn and different side effects of heartburn.

High fat dinners and broiled food sources

Greasy food sources by and large lower tension on your LES and defer stomach exhausting. This might build your gamble for reflux side effects, as per the National Institute of Diabetes and Digestive and Kidney Diseases.

To assist with forestalling reflux, you can take a stab at diminishing your all out fat admission.

Here are a few high fat food varieties you might need to keep away from:

french fries

rotisserie onion rings

potato chips

margarine

entire milk

cheddar

frozen yogurt

high fat harsh cream

high fat velvety plate of mixed greens dressings

velvety sauces and plunges

high fat cuts of red meat, like marbled sirloin or prime rib

For instance, you might encounter side effects in the wake of consuming:

chocolate

mint, like peppermint or spearmint

vigorously handled food varieties

anti-toxins

ibuprofen or other pain killers

bisphosphonates

alpha-blockers

nitrates

calcium channel blockers

tricyclics

theophylline

iron or potassium supplements

You might be enticed to quit taking a drug or supplement on the off chance that you believe it's rising your indigestion or indigestion side effects.

Chapter 17: Indigestion, Acid Reflux, Or

Gerd?

I

n some cases different words are utilized to allude to acid reflux, similar to heartburn or GERD. Yet, they don't all mean exactly the same thing. To treat indigestion, understanding the difference is useful.

Indigestion is a side effect. It implies the sensation of consuming agony in your chest. The aggravation ordinarily fires behind your breastbone and climbs toward your throat.

Heartburn happens when your stomach corrosive ventures too high up in your stomach related framework. Typically, gravity and your stomach related framework cooperate to hold stomach corrosive down in your stomach where it should be. Be that as it may, some of the time it can ascend into your throat and cause disturbance, acid reflux, or different side effects.

You could have known about GERD — it's a more limited name for gastroesophageal reflux infection. While this condition can have various causes and side effects, it frequently includes acid reflux. GERD can at times prompt serious confusions, so in the event that you have indigestion as often as possible, talk with a specialist.

How normal is acid reflux?

Incidental acid reflux is genuinely normal. In any case, in the event that you have normal and extreme acid reflux, it very well may be a mark of a constant heartburn condition called GERD. You ought to converse with your medical services supplier assuming you much of the time experience acid reflux.

What does indigestion feel like?

Indigestion normally feels like a consuming in the focal point of your chest, behind your breastbone. At the point when you have indigestion, you may likewise feel side effects like:

•A consuming inclination in chest that is capable to endure anyplace from a couple of moments to two or more hours.

•Torment in your chest when you twist around or set down.

131

•A consuming inclination in your throat.

•A hot, harsh, acidic, or pungent desire for the rear of your throat.

•Trouble gulping.

Potential Causes

What causes acid reflux?

To know why acid reflux occurs, it can assist with understanding how your throat and stomach work. At the point when you eat, the food passes down a long cylinder that interfaces your mouth and stomach. This cylinder is known as the throat. At the lower part of the throat is a valve, called the esophageal sphincter. This valve opens to let food through and afterward closes to keep your stomach contents down. Inside your stomach is an exceptionally impressive acidic blend that begins the most common way of separating your food (processing). Your stomach is intended to hold this combination. Notwithstanding, your throat can't hold this combination without getting injured.

Once in a while, the valve that isolates your stomach and throat doesn't close as expected, and a portion of the acidic combinations from your stomach return up the throat. This is called reflux. At the point when you have reflux, you'll frequently feel the consuming vibe that is indigestion. There are a couple of ailments that can cause reflux and cause you to feel indigestion, including:

•Pregnancy.

•Hiatal hernia

•Gastroesophageal reflux illness (GERD).

•Certain meds, particularly calming medications and headache medicine.

Indigestion can likewise be brought about by your dietary patterns — including the food sources you eat, how huge your dinners are, and how near sleep time you eat — and certain way of life propensities.

What can set off acid reflux?

Indigestion can be set off by a wide range of things that are a piece of your day to day existence. For some individuals, indigestion can be brought about by specific eating and way of life propensities. These propensities can include things like eating huge segments of food, eating excessively near sleep time, or in any event, having high-feelings of anxiety.

Certain food varieties and beverages can likewise set off indigestion for certain individuals. A few food varieties and beverages that could set off your indigestion can include:

•Onions.

•Citrus natural products.

•High-fat food sources.

•Tomatoes.

•Tomato-based items.

•Liquor.

•Citrus juices.

•Jazzed drinks.

•Carbonated refreshments.

Your way of life propensities can likewise have an impact in why you could encounter indigestion. These regular factors frequently add to ailments that cause acid reflux, as GERD or hiatal hernia. Some way of life propensities that can set off your indigestion include:

•Being overweight.

•Being a smoker.

•Having a high-anxiety.

•Wearing tight garments and belts.

Chapter 18: Care And Treatment

How is acid reflux treated?

M

uch of the time, acid reflux can be treated at home with non-prescription drugs and changes to way of life propensities that cause the inclination. Intermittent acid reflux is normal and is ordinarily not serious. In any case, assuming you have continuous and serious acid reflux, connect with your medical services supplier. This could be an indication of a persistent condition like GERD. GERD can prompt other serious infections like esophagitis, Barrett's throat, and even malignant growth. Once in a while, your PCP might maintain that should do an endoscopy to check for fundamental drug conditions. An endoscopy is the assessment of your gastrointestinal system with a lit adaptable instrument.

Non-prescription meds for indigestion regularly incorporate stomach settling agents and corrosive blockers.

How do stomach settling agents work to treat indigestion?

Stomach settling agents diminish how much stomach corrosive, alleviating your indigestion. These drugs can likewise be utilized to relieve stomach upset, heartburn, and different agonies in your stomach. A few acid neutralizers contain simethicone, which lessens gas. Stomach settling agents that you can get without a solution include:

•Tums®.

•Rolaids®.

•Maalox®.

Ensure you generally adhere to the guidelines on the bundle or converse with your primary care physician about the correct method for utilizing an acid neutralizer. Assuming that you use tablets, bite them a long time prior to gulping them for quicker help.

Are there any results of stomach settling agents?

A few stomach settling agents contain magnesium or sodium bicarbonate, which can carry on like a diuretic. Try not to take acid neutralizers assuming you have any side effects of an infected appendix or entrail aggravation. Results of stomach settling agents might include:

•Clogging.

•Looseness of the bowels.

•White or pale defecations.

•Stomach cramps.

Serious secondary effects can happen with an excess or abuse of acid neutralizers.

How do corrosive blockers attempt to treat acid reflux?

Items like Pepcid AC® are called receptor H2 blockers, or corrosive blockers. Corrosive blockers lessen the development of stomach corrosive. They assuage acid reflux, corrosive heartburn, and acrid stomach. Continuously follow the bearings on the bundling or converse with your medical services supplier about how to take this drug. Corrosive blockers you can purchase without a solution include:

• Pepcid AC®.

• Tagamet HB®.

Take your corrosive blocker medication consistently however long coordinated by your medical services supplier, regardless of whether you have any aggravation or on the other hand on the off chance that your side effects improve.

More powerful corrosive blockers are physician endorsed meds. These can be utilized to obstruct stomach corrosive, treat stomach and duodenal ulcers, erosive esophagitis, and GERD. They work by decreasing the development of stomach corrosive. Your medical care supplier will give you a particular remedy for this sort of corrosive blocker.

The United States Food and Drug Administration (FDA) as of late revealed raised levels of a potential cancer-causing agent, NDMA, in the medications ranitidine (Zantac®) and nizatidine (Axid®). You ought to address your medical services supplier assuming you are taking one of these meds.

Are there any symptoms of corrosive blockers?

Symptoms of corrosive blockers include:

• Migraine.

• Unsteadiness.

• The runs.

In the event that you have any of the accompanying conceivably serious secondary effects subsequent to taking corrosive blockers, tell your medical services supplier immediately:

• Disarray.

• Chest snugness.

• Dying.

• Sore throat.

• Fever.

• Sporadic heartbeat.

• Shortcoming or surprising weariness.

Would it be a good idea for me to take stomach settling agents and corrosive blockers together to treat indigestion?

Your medical services supplier might believe you should accept stomach settling agents while taking corrosive blockers. Stomach settling agents will control your side effects until the corrosive blockers begin to work. In the event that your primary care physician recommends a stomach settling agent, take it an hour prior (or an hour later) you take a corrosive blocker.

Chapter 19: What Are Doctor Prescribed

Meds For Acid Reflux?

I

n the event that over-the-counter stomach settling agents and corrosive blockers don't ease your indigestion, your medical services supplier might give you a solution for different meds, for example,

•Original effectiveness corrosive blockers: In original potency (normally higher portions), Zantac®, Tagamet®, Pepcid®, and Axid® can by and large alleviate acid reflux and treat GERD.

•Proton siphon inhibitors: These are drugs that block corrosive creation all the more successfully. Proton siphon inhibitors incorporate Aciphex®, Nexium®, Prevacid®, Prilosec®, and Protonix®.

Some proton siphon inhibitors can be bought over the counter. Converse with your medical care supplier about these prescriptions and what is best for you.

Could I at any point forestall acid reflux?

You can frequently forestall and oversee acid reflux by making changes to your eating routine and way of life. These progressions include:

•Not heading to sleep with a full stomach. Eat feasts somewhere around three to four hours before you rests. This gives your stomach time to exhaust and lessens the possibility encountering indigestion short-term.

•Abstaining from gorging. Scaling back the size of your bits during dinners can assist with bringing down your gamble of indigestion. You can likewise have a go at eating four or five little feasts rather than three bigger ones.

•Dialing back. Eating gradually can frequently assist with forestalling acid reflux. Put your fork down among chomps and abstain from eating excessively fast.

•Wearing baggy garments. Belts and tight apparel can some of the time cause acid reflux. By changing your closet to stay away from these things, you could possibly forestall having indigestion.

•Keeping away from specific food varieties. For some individuals, certain food varieties trigger acid reflux. Staying away from these food sources can help. Have a go at keeping a log of these food sources so you can look out for them later on. Your medical services supplier may likewise recommend that you stay away from liquor.

•Keeping a sound weight. Getting thinner can frequently assist with alleviating acid reflux.

•Not smoking. Nicotine can debilitate the lower esophageal sphincter (the valve that isolates your stomach and throat). Not smoking is suggested for your overall wellbeing, as well as the strength of this valve.

•Resting on your left side. This might help absorption and the expulsion of corrosive from your stomach and throat all the more rapidly.

•Raising the top of your bed with the goal that your head and chest are higher than your feet. Place 6-inch blocks or books under the bed posts at the top of the bed. Try not to utilize heaps of pads. They might make you put more squeeze on your stomach and aggravate your acid reflux.

•Arranging your activity to stay away from acid reflux. Stand by no less than two hours after a dinner prior to working out. Assuming you sort out any sooner, you might set off acid reflux. You ought to likewise drink a lot of water previously and during exercise. Water helps processing and forestalls lack of hydration.

When to Call the Doctor

When would it be advisable for me to call my primary care physician about my acid reflux?

Despite the fact that acid reflux is normal, it can some of the time lead to more serious medical conditions. Extreme, ongoing indigestion has been connected to irritation and restricting of the throat, respiratory issues, persistent hack, GERD, and Barrett's throat, which might prompt esophageal malignant growth.

You ought to contact your primary care physician if:

•Your acid reflux will not disappear.

•Your indigestion side effects become more serious or incessant.

•It's hard or damages to swallow.

145

•Your indigestion makes you upchuck.

•You have had significant, unforeseen weight reduction.

•You assume control over-the-counter acid neutralizers for over two weeks (or for a more extended time frame than suggested on the mark) you actually have indigestion side effects.

•You have indigestion side effects even subsequent to taking professionally prescribed meds.

•You have serious dryness or wheezing.

•Your distress slows down your way of life or day to day exercises.

Will indigestion disappear all alone?

For some individuals, intermittent acid reflux is normal. By watching what you eat and staying away from specific triggers (diet and way of life propensities), you might have the option to forestall acid reflux or oversee it. Assuming you find that you much of the time experience indigestion and that it continues to deteriorate, it very well may be an indication of an ailment like GERD. In these cases, your acid reflux will not leave without treatment. Converse with your medical services supplier so you can foster a therapy plan.

Chapter 20: Food Varieties That Fight

Heartburn

Y

ou've caught wind of the food sources that can aggravate your indigestion, from espresso to chocolate to tomatoes. Yet, shouldn't something be said about food varieties that could improve your acid reflux? Look at some key eats you ought to add to your eating regimen.

Eat More Low-Acid Foods

At the point when corrosive and different fluids in your stomach back up into your throat, you get acid reflux. However, the corrosive that is now in your stomach isn't the main issue.

The regular acids in food varieties you eat - - in the same way as other natural products, vegetables, and beverages. To control indigestion, fabricate your feasts around normally low-corrosive food varieties like:

•Melons and bananas. While most natural products have a high corrosive substance, these don't. Bananas are generally helpful as a nibble food. A wide range of melons are great, similar to watermelon, melon, and honeydew.

•Cereal. Cereal doesn't cause reflux, it's filling, and it has bunches of sound fiber.

•Bread. Pick entire grain - - it will be the principal fixing on the mark - - which is made with natural grains. Other solid sounding bread - - like wheat, entire wheat, or 7-grain - - might be made with refined grains, which are deprived of regular fiber, nutrients, and different supplements.

•Rice and couscous. These solid complex carbs are perfect assuming that you have reflux. While picking rice, go for earthy colored rice, which has more fiber.

•Green veggies. Broccoli, asparagus, green beans, celery, and cauliflower are low in corrosive.

•Lean poultry and meats. Get ready chicken and turkey barbecued, cooked, prepared, or steamed. Simply eliminate the skin - - and don't broil it, Roland says. Indeed, even ground hamburger and steak can be fine, for however long they're lean.

•Potatoes. Other root vegetables are great, as well - - simply not onions.

•Fish. Barbecued, poached, and prepared fish are great decisions. Simply don't sear it or utilize greasy sauces.

•Egg whites. They're a decent wellspring of protein and are low in corrosive. Simply skirt the yolk, which is bound to cause side effects.

You can't perceive how acidic a food is by checking it out. It's not on the sustenance mark by the same token. In any case, you can explore a food's pH, which is a score of its corrosive substance. The lower the pH number, the higher the corrosive - - lemon juice has a pH of 2.0. In the event that you go for the gold a pH of 5 or above, you might have less side effects. You can find the pH level of food sources on some administration destinations and in low-corrosive eating regimen cookbooks.

More Foods to Soothe Heartburn

Different food sources and spices have for quite some time been medicines for reflux and upset stomachs. In any case, remember that while they might give alleviation to certain, "they won't work for everybody," should attempt:

•Fennel. This crunchy vegetable with a licorice flavor makes an incredible expansion to plates of mixed greens. There's some proof that fennel can work on your absorption. It has a pH of 6.9, so it's low in corrosive, as well.

•Ginger. A well-established regular treatment for upset stomachs, ginger appears to have benefits for reflux.

•Parsley. That twig of parsley on your plate isn't just for enrichment. Parsley has been a conventional treatment for upset stomachs for many years.

•Aloe vera. This is one more old treatment for GI issues that appears to assist with reflux. You can purchase aloe vera as a plant or as an enhancement - - in containers, juices, and different structures. It fills in as a thickener in recipes. Simply ensure it's liberated from anthraquinones (essentially the compound aloin), which can be aggravating to the stomach related framework.

Chapter 21: Battle Heartburn With Healthy

Food

A

dd the right food sources to your eating regimen. They could assist with your acid reflux. Yet, there are points to what they can reach.

Recall that great food can't check the impacts of trigger food sources. "Eating somewhat ginger won't prevent you from getting indigestion after a major supper of a greasy steak, a serving of mixed greens with tomatoes, two or three glasses of wine, and an espresso,".

And keeping in mind that eating a low-corrosive eating routine is a decent technique, it may not be enough all alone. For certain individuals, it's not such a lot of the acids in the stomach, yet the reflux of other stuff in gastric juices - - like bile - - that trigger indigestion, he says.

"The particular reasons for indigestion fluctuate a ton from one individual to another,". "That is the reason treatment in every case needs a customized approach."

How is acid reflux analyzed?

A specialist by and large judgments indigestion in light of your side effects and clinical history. During the arrangement when you're analyzed, your primary care physician can suggest a treatment plan.

You might have to see your medical care proficient once more assuming way of life changes, OTC medicine, or physician endorsed drug don't work on your side effects. This might be an indication that you have a more difficult condition called GERD.

To analyze GERD, your PCP will audit your clinical history and get some information about your side effects. They may likewise arrange a few tests, including:

•Walking corrosive (pH) test. Your PCP will pass a little cylinder through your nose into your throat. A sensor at the tip of the cylinder estimates how much stomach corrosive in your throat.

•Esophageal pH checking. Your PCP puts a case on the coating of your throat to quantify heartburn.

•X-beam. You'll drink a white fluid that covers your upper intestinal system. Your PCP will then utilize X-beam imaging to take a gander at your throat, stomach, and upper digestive tract.

•Endoscopy. Your primary care physician will pass a little cylinder outfitted with a camera down your throat into your stomach to check for a ulcer of the throat or stomach lining.

•Esophageal manometry. Your PCP will put a cylinder through your nose into your throat to gauge the constrictions of your throat when you swallow.

Contingent upon your conclusion, your PCP will actually want to furnish you with treatment choices to help lessen or kill your side effects.

What are the inconveniences related with acid reflux?

Intermittent indigestion isn't regularly a reason to worry. Notwithstanding, successive indigestion might be a side effect of GERD. This condition might require treatment with physician endorsed prescription or medical procedure.

Whenever left untreated, GERD might prompt extra medical conditions, for example, an aggravation of the throat, which is called esophagitis, or Barrett's throat. Barrett's throat causes changes in the covering of the throat that can build your gamble of esophageal disease.

Long haul indigestion can likewise influence your personal satisfaction. See your PCP decide a course of treatment on the off chance that you find it hard to carry on your regular routine or are seriously restricted in your exercises because of indigestion.

Food sources to Avoid to Prevent Heartburn

The greater part of indigestion victims taking drugs feel not exactly happy with their outcomes (per a new Gallup overview). Luckily, there are many solutions for indigestion other than basically venturing into the medication bureau; only a couple of diet changes might be sufficient to avert the red hot sensation. However it particularly relies upon the individual, a few normal trigger food sources will generally influence many individuals and might worth keep away from.

- Liquor
- Espresso and other energized food and drink
- Carbonated drinks
- Zesty food sources
- Onions
- Citrus leafy foods
- Mint
- Tomatoes and tomato items
- Huge, greasy, as well as seared feasts

Chapter 22: Physiological Factors:

Pregnancy:

During pregnancy most of the females have complain of heartburn. The reason for this is that pregnancy alters the normal hormonal level in body. The secretion of progesterone is very high. Progesterone has relaxing effect on smooth muscle cells. It not only relaxes the smooth muscles of uterus bus also brings about the relaxation of lower esophageal sphincter. This keeps the sphincter relaxed for longer duration promoting the acid reflux. Other effects of progesterone include decreased intestinal motility due the relaxation of smooth muscles of gut. The intestinal contents move slowly and stomach gets full. This leads to gastric reflux and mother starts feeling nauseatic.

Other reason for heartburn during pregnancy is that during trimester the fetus grows rapidly and weight gain is very prominent. Till the birth the child continues to increase in both weight and size. Now more space is required to accommodate the fetus. So the growing placenta and fetus try to occupy more space in mother's abdomen thus pressing against the intestine and push the stomach upward. This compression of stomach reduces its storage capacity and stomach tries to get rid of its contents whenever it is full i.e. when the meal is taken. This promotes vomiting and acid reflux in pregnant females.

Nutritional factors:

The importance of food and nutrition cannot be denied in case of heartburn. Sometimes the fault lies within our diet. We start consuming food which triggers the acid release and becomes the culprit for heartburn.

When fatty or protein food enters the stomach it stimulates the production of hormone "gastrin". Gastrin is the potent stimulus for the production of gastric juice and acid. Along with acid production the function of gastrin is to strengthen the contractions of stomach and lower the tone of lower esophageal sphincter. So increased gastrin production is also responsible for gastric reflux. There are many foods which stimulate the production of gastrin and are the causative agents for heartburn.

Alcohols:

Alcohols stimulate the acid production. The mechanism of action is through increased gastrin production. That is why alcohols are dangerous for life and serious consequences are seen.

Caffeine:

Caffeine is the active ingredients of tea and coffee. People who consume too much tea or coffee often suffer from gastric problems such acidity and heartburn because caffeine increases the hcl production.

Beverages:

Soft drinks and beverages contain acidic products which stimulate acid production and relax lower esophageal sphincter.

Spicy food:

Chilies, food flavors, spicy food also promote the acid production and reflux. Actually

Spices stimulate the cephalic phase of acid secretion (phase during which even the smell or sight or food starts producing hcl). The vagal nerves are responsible for this because vagal nerves supply to stomach is stimulatory. When a person has sight or smell of food it increases vagal discharge and ultimately the more acid is produced.

Fried foods:

The major cause of heartburn in modern era is junk food. We people are so used to them these days without knowing the consequences. Fried foods put pressure on stomach and prolong the relaxation of lower esophageal sphincter.

Citrus juices:

Intake of citrus juices increases the production of gastric acid and cause acidity.

Large meals:

Overeating is one the most common causes of gastric acid production. Lying down after taking large meal should be avoided as this will put pressure on weak lower esophageal sphincter thus relaxing it.

Fatty food:

Consuming fatty food distends the stomach and forces the lower esophageal sphincter to relax the food is pushed back. Fats in fact decrease the production of hcl but when they reach small intestine a hormone " enterogestrone" is released. The function of this hormone is to inhibit the secretion of gastrin release from stomach and delaying the gastric emptying. The reason is that gastrin is needed for the gastric emptying so when gastrin is inhibited the gastric emptying will also be slowed down.

High protein diet:

Main function of stomach is to digest protein by secreting gastric juice containing many enzymes. So whenever the protein intake is higher the secretion of gastric juice increases. Overproduction of gastric juice is dangerous because enzymes in this juice start digesting the stomach walls. It turns out to be the cause of pain and heartburn.

Pathological factors:

Many pathological factors and diseases associated with abnormality of lower esophageal sphincter are responsible for causing gastric reflux and heartburn.

Abnormal anti-reflux barrier:

Anti-reflux barrier provides resistance to gastric reflux. The components of this barrier are lower esophageal sphincter, cruras of diaphragms and esophageal ligaments. Lower esophageal sphincter is under the control of neural and hormonal mechanisms. It has myogenic activity and its tonic contractions provide the protection against gastric reflux. Usually the sphincter remains contracted and provides the barrier between esophagus and stomach. It relaxes only when a person eats and bolus of food is pushed downward through peristaltic activity. Relaxation also occurs in response to gastric distention for the purpose of air venting.

Now we fully understand the importance of lower esophageal system in preventing the gastric reflux. Any abnormalities in it make the person more prone to regurgitation of gastric contents. The length of this sphincter is the criteria for judging its functional capability.

Length of lower esophageal sphincter:

A pressure gradient is developed between the low pressure zone in thoracic cavity and high pressure zone in abdomen. Lower esophageal sphincter is the area of high pressure. It must be able to resist the increase in intra-abdominal and intra-gastric pressure. The abdominal part of sphincter is subjected to high pressure so its competency is estimated by its power to resist the increase in pressure. The greater the tonic contraction of the sphincter stronger will be the anti-reflux barrier. In addition to tonic contractions the reflux contractions of diaphragmatic cruras maintains the integrity of the barrier. It is important to know that length of this sphincter determines its strength and its ability to prevent the high gastric pressure. The overall length should be adequate for the proper functioning of the lower esophageal sphincter. If the length is proper then any rise in gastric or abdominal pressure can be resisted. But in the persons with short length of this sphincter the gastric reflux is more common. 60% to 70% of the patients with the GERD disease have the mechanical deficiency of lower esophageal sphincter.

Position of lower esophageal sphincter:

After the length the position of lower esophageal sphincter is also important for its functioning. The part of the sphincter that resists the increase in gastric pressure must be located within abdominal part of esophagus. If a large portion of this sphincter is present within abdominal part of esophagus then it will have more tendencies to collapse when the gastric pressure rises.

When the gastric pressure increases the abdominal part of lower esophageal sphincter contracts. Simultaneously the diaphragm also contracts facilitating the closure of sphincter. Thus the gastric reflux is prevented.

Impaired esophageal clearance:

Esophageal clearance is the second major protective mechanism against gastric reflux. Esophageal clearance means the rate at which the acid is cleared from esophagus. Abnormality in esophageal clearance results in repeated exposure of esophagus to acid causing damage to esophageal epithelium. Esophageal clearance is a two step process. First there is esophageal emptying followed by acid neutralization. Esophageal emptying is prompted by peristaltic waves while acid neutralization is done by salivation. There are four factors which promote the esophageal clearance. These are:

Peristaltic contractions:

Peristaltic waves are the rhythmic contractions of gastrointestinal tracts starting from esophagus towards anus. These contractions make the intestinal contents to move. Primary role during esophageal clearance is done by peristaltic contractions. When the bolus of food passes through esophagus the nervous control takes over and the peristaltic contractions are initiated. Major portion of gastric juice and acid is cleared by these peristaltic contractions. These contractions are of two types; primary and secondary peristalsis. Primary peristalsis is initiated by swallowing centre when the bolus of food reaches esophagus. They last for 8-10 seconds. These are the strong contractions and provide the major protective mechanism against gastric reflux. If the acid residues are left in the esophagus this initiates the secondary peristaltic contractions which remove the remaining food materials. This type of clearance is also called "volume clearance". As long as the peristaltic contractions are normal the esophagus remains cleared of food contents and acid. But in any case if the motor activity of esophagus gets impaired the peristaltic contractions are slowed down. Food stays for longer time in esophagus and regurgitation

Salivation:

Salivation helps in esophageal clearance by neutralizing acid in esophagus. This happens when the intra-esophageal pH falls. Fall in pH stimulates the salivation and more saliva is produced to neutralize the acid. Proper salivation is very important because it provides protection against the adverse affects of acid. Saliva restores the acidic pH of esophagus back to normal. Reduced saliva production increases the time for clearance. But if the salivation is stimulated the time taken for esophageal salivation gets shorter. Studies have shown that sucking lozenges stimulate salivation and improves the clearance. Clearance by the help of salivation is called "chemical clearance"

Gravity:

Gravity aids the esophageal clearance by forcing the downward movement of food through the esophagus. Usually in normal persons the gravity does not play any significant role in acid clearance however in patients with GERD disease or with impaired motor activity, gravity becomes an important factor. It is advised for such patients to lie with the head raised off the bed as this will maintain the gravity and helps in keeping the esophagus cleared.

Position of distal part of esophagus:

Distal part of esophagus contains lower esophageal sphincter which prevents the acid reflux. The position of distal part is significant in this perspective. If the lower part of esophagus is located within abdomen it will be able to resist the pressure changes in stomach. Any upward displacement in position makes the sphincter weak and promotes the gastric reflux.

☐   Increased abdominal pressure:

Most of the obese people complain about heartburn. In this case the culprit is obesity itself. Obese is nothing else but the accumulation of excess fats in body. The abdominal tissues have more tendencies to store extra fats. So when a person puts on weight abdomen is the first part where fats start accumulating. Consequences are drastic. Along with other clinical symptoms the person becomes more prone towards gastric acid reflux. Actually the fat storage leads to increased abdominal pressure and this put more pressure on stomach. Now the peristaltic movements are not enough to resist this pressure. So the downward propulsive movements, which normally cause the movement of food throughout the gastrointestinal tract, are disrupted. High pressure pushes the food and acid in stomach in upward direction. As a result gastric reflux starts producing the sensation of heartburn.

Weight put on depends on our lifestyle. In modern age when everyone is running out of time there is no spare time for walk or exercise. We usually sit or lie down after meals. The food does not get proper time to reach the stomach. So the acid reflux starts. That is why it is advised to walk after having meal or sit in upright posture for at least 45 min. This will improve the gastric motility and digestion.

☐   Duodenal-gastric reflux:

This is different from gastro-esophageal reflux in which acid regurgitates into esophagus. In duodenal gastric reflux the biliary fluid moves into stomach and esophagus. This is also called "biliary reflux". Stomach consists of pyloric sphincter at its distal end. It is a powerful sphincter which controls the gastric emptying. This sphincter also prevents the backward movement of duodenal contents into stomach. Biliary reflux is common in people with the abnormality or weakness of pyloric sphincter. Usually the patients after the gastric surgery complain of dyspepsia and heartburn. In these patients the pyloric sphincter gets weakened. This promotes the backward movement of duodenal contents into stomach. Effects of this reflux are serious. It damages the gastric mucosa causing its hyperemia. This reflux causes:

-    Gastritis

169

- Esophageal carcinoma

- Antral ulcers

- Barrett's esophagus (metaplasic change; stratified squamous epithelium of esophagus is replaced by columnar epithelium)

☐ Delayed gastric emptying:

Stomach is the hollow, muscular organ of digestion especially of proteins. When the bolus of food reaches the stomach it is pushed downwards towards the duodenum. Movement of food through stomach is controlled by peristaltic contractions. The rhythmic peristaltic contractions start from the cardiac end of stomach towards its pyloric end. The peristalsis is under the control of hormonal and neural mechanisms.

Motor activity of stomach:

- Parasympathetic system increases the gastrointestinal motility.

- Sympathetic system supplies the sphincter. The sympathetic supply to pyloric sphincter keeps it contracted. It opens only when the stomach has to empty its contents.

170

Hormonal mechanisms:

There are many hormones which either promote or inhibit the gastric emptying:

-    Gastrin stimulates emptying

-    Chlosystokinin inhibits emptying

-    Motilin increases gastric motility

-    Gastric inhibitory polypeptide delays emptying

Factors promoting delayed gastric emptying:

Distention of duodenal walls:

When the chyme from the stomach enters duodenum it stretches the walls of duodenum. This stretching initiates a reflux known as " Enterogastric Reflux". It is an inhibitory mechanism. This reflux inhibits the parasympathetic discharge and in turn decreases gastrin production. As a result the gastric peristalsis slow down thus prolongs gastric emptying. But at the same time sympathetic activity increases which keeps the pyloric sphincter in contracted state. Thus this mechanism inhibits gastric emptying and promotes gastric reflux.

171

Chapter 24: Foods To Avoid During

Heartburn

Many foods trigger the release of gastric acid. So diet plays an important role in regulating the gastric acid secretion. A bit change in diet plan can be really helpful for relieving the symptoms of heartburn. Following foods should be avoided during GERD:

☐   Avoid fried foods:

Fried food delays the stomach emptying and is retained in stomach for longer time. This stimulates the production of gastric acid. So the French fries lovers are suggested to think before eating fried foods because these foods might cause heartburn and bloating.

☐   Avoids meat products:

Meat products stimulate the gastric acid production. People who frequently take meat in diets complain of acid reflux and heartburn. So patients with the GERD should avoid meat products like ground beef, chicken nuggets, and chicken wings.

☐   Avoid fatty foods:

Fatty foods are not easily digestible. They stay for longer time in stomach. More acid is produced to digest it. Fatty food puts pressure on lower esophageal sphincter thus relaxing it. Acid reflux is common in people who are fond of junk food like burgers and pizzas because these foods have high fat content. So it advised to avoid junk food as much as possible.

☐ Avoid citrus fruits:

Although citrus fruits are the major source of vitamin C but their excess consumption can cause acid reflux and heartburn. Citrus fruits contain citrus acid which irritates the gastric mucosa and stimulates the production of gastric acid.

☐ Avoid soft drinks and beverages:

Excess use of beverages is not good for the health. These are the acid containing drinks and act as irritant for stomach. They increase the hcl production promoting acid reflux. So use of soft drinks and beverages should be limited.

☐ Avoid coffee and tea:

Excess of everything is bad. People who take a lot of coffee and tea everyday must limit it. Coffee and tea contain caffeine which a stimulant for gastric acid release. So try to avoid coffee and tea because they often produce the symptoms of heartburn.

☐   Avoid chocolates:

Well everyone lives to eat chocolates but chocolates can be the cause of heartburn and acid reflux. Their active ingredient is caffeine which stimulates the acid production by stomach. So avoid chocolates if you feel heartburn after their consumption.

☐   Avoid milk products:

Dairy products like cream, milk shakes and cottage cheese should be avoided because they contain fat and are not easy to digest. These produce often produce excess gas and cause bloating, nausea and heartburn.

☐   Avoid spicy foods:

Spicy food has become the trend now but we should also know the consequences of spicy food. Use of excess chilies, spices and peppermint in food can be injurious for your stomach health. These are the irritants and stimulants for the release of gastric acid. Too much consumption of spicy food causes heartburn and acid reflux.

☐   Avoid grains:

Use of grains like macaronis, beans and wheat products should be limited. Some people are sensitive to wheat products because they contain gluten which irritates the stomach. As a result more acid is produced. It does not mean that you can never eat these products but a balanced should be maintained.

☐   Avoid alcohols:

Beware alcohol consumers. Alcohol is a very strong irritant and injurious for the stomach. It has and erosive action on gastric mucosa and the production of gastric acid is potentiated by its use. So the acid reflux starts. In severe cases it can lead to peptic ulcers as well.

FOODS TO BE TAKEN DURING HEARTBURN:

☐   Oat meals:

Oats are the best option during GERD and heartburn. They are easily digestible and

175

prevent the acidity in stomach. It is advised for the patients of GERD to take oats in breakfast.

☐ **Ginger:**

If you are suffering from heartburn and acid reflux then add some ginger to your food. Studies have shown that ginger has anti-inflammatory properties. It saves the gastric mucosa from the adverse effects of acid. Apart from anti-inflammatory action it also adds a good flavor to food.

☐ **Pasta:**

Pasta is another alternative food for the patients of heartburn because it contains high fiber and is easily digestible. But avoid the use of tomato sauces and chilies with pasta. Try to eat it with the mixture of fresh vegetables.

☐ Sea foods:

Sea foods for example fish is the recommended diet for the patients of heartburn because they contain fewer calories as compared to beef and mutton and produce less amount of gastric acid. So sea foods are good for heartburn.

☐ **Salads:**

Fresh salads without cream dressing are very effective for the heartburn patients. They combat the acidity produced in stomach. Salads soothe the gastric lining and reduce the release of gastric acid.

☐ **Fruits:**

Fruits with high fiber content must be taken during cases of acid reflux. These fruits reduce the secretion of gastric therefore the chances of hear burn are lessened. Apples, bananas, peaches, pears, melon are fiber rich fruits.

☐ **Beans:**

Patients of GERD are advised not to take the meat products. But the question arises that from where will they get proteins then? Answer is here. Beans are the best alternatives of meat. They are rich in proteins and amino acids. On the other hand they can be digested easily and reduce the acid release. So must add beans to your diet if want to get rid of symptoms of heartburn and gastric acidity.

☐ Whole grains:

Whole grains are rich in fibers. Fibers are very effective for counteracting the acidity and heartburn. Fibers add bulk to the food and give the feeling of fullness. They increase the motility of gastrointestinal tract and increase the gastric emptying as well. Food is not allowed to stay in stomach for loner duration so the less acid is produced and the chances of gastric and acid reflux are reduced. Eat whole wheat bread, brown rice, oats, and cereals to get rid of heartburn.

☐ **Vegetables:**

Try to eat fresh and leafy vegetables because they contain fibers in them. Fibers increase the gastric motility and aid in the process of digestion. Raw vegetables have alkaline nature. They can neutralize the excess acid produced in stomach. They also contain certain enzymes which help in digestion. That is why is advised to eat raw or lightly cooked vegetable. Overcooking destroys the enzymes so their effectiveness is reduced.

☐ Potassium rich food:

Potassium is responsible for the smooth muscles contractions. And we know that the cause of acid reflux is the abnormality of lower esophageal sphincter. The sphincter is unable to contract properly. Potassium rich foods will help in this case. They increase the contractility of lower esophageal sphincter to some extent and prevent the back splash of acid into esophagus. So potassium rich diets for example banana, apple cider vinegar, apples and sweet potatoes are suggested for the GERD patients.

☐   Drink water:

Drink plenty of water to avoid the acidity. At least 8-10 glasses of water are necessary. If you drink a lot of water it will keep your stomach cleared of the acid and reduces the chances of acid reflux.

☐   Fresh juices:

Take fresh juices like apple juice. They not only provide the essential nutrients and vitamins but also reduce the gastric acid secretion. But avoid the citrus juices like orange and lemon juice because they aggravate the acidity.

☐   **Milk:**

Milk is effective against acidity. It neutralizes the excess acid and also regulates its production. So drink a glass of milk before bed time to prevent acidity.

179

LIFESTYLE CHANGES:

In most of the cases reason of heartburn and acidity is our lifestyle. Our routine activities and habits decide the physical health. Now no one has time to pay attention to their daily schedule. That is why acidity has become the common problem now days. Everyone should follow some simple steps to avoid acidity and heartburn.

☐   Take small meals:

Take small meals instead of 3 big meals per day. Big meals distend the stomach and cause the release of more acid. Also they put pressure on lower esophageal sphincter causing its relaxation and promoting the gastric reflux. Take frequent meals and add vegetables and fruits to the diet.

☐   Take big meals in lunch:

It is fine if you take big meal in lunch time because heavy meal at night time leads to the overnight production of gastric acid even during sleep. This can be really painful and the sleep of the person is also affected. So avoid large meals at night.

☐   Take meal 2-3 hours before bedtime:

180

Our eating habits are so irregular. In most of the time we take meal just before the bed time. So stop doing this. It is advised to take your meal at least 2 to 3 hours before going to bed. This time gap is necessary if you want to avoid the heartburn because during this time the stomach completes its digestion and gets cleared of the acid produced during digestion. So change your eating habits and see the good results.

☐   Do not lie down after taking meal:

Again the culprit is our lifestyle. Lying down immediately after taking meal leads to acidity, heartburn and nausea. We love to eat and sleep. But seriously we are causing harm to ourselves. When you lie down after taking the meal, pressure on stomach is increased the gastric contents are pressed against the lower esophageal sphincter. The sphincter gets relaxed and the gastric reflux starts. So it is advised not to lie down immediately after the meal.

☐   Do not overeat:

Overeating contributes to heartburn and gastric reflux. Many people are food lovers. They never get conscious about their eating habits. But they should be aware of the consequences also because overeating does only harm to the body. When you do overeating the stomach gets stuffed and the food is pushed upwards towards the lower esophageal sphincter forcing it to relax. Relaxation of lower esophageal sphincter allows the food to regurgitate back into esophagus. That is why everyone can experience heartburn, acidity and dyspepsia.

☐ Avoid late night snacks:

Once you are in bed at night try to avoid eating anything. The late night snacks trigger the release of acid from stomach. The stomach will need time to get cleared of its contents. So if you sleep after taking snacks it will be a discomfort for you because as long as the acid remains in stomach it keeps on irritating the gastric mucosa and the symptoms of heartburn appear.

☐ Do not eat quickly:

When you eat quickly the stomach is unable to digest the food completely so fast. As a result more and more acid is produced to aid the digestion. Quick eating leads to the entrapping of excess air in stomach causing its distention. Gastric distention has two effects:

-    It promotes the acid production.

-    Excess air in stomach causes bloating and gastric reflux and farting

There are few ways and steps to avoid the fast eating:

-    Relax while eating

-    Chew food properly

-    Take smaller bites because they are easy to digest.

☐   Lose weight:

Obesity increases the risk of gastric reflux and heartburn. Obese people more often suffer from the heartburn and acidity. Obesity increases the abdominal compression. It puts pressure on stomach. When the stomach is compressed its contents are pushed against the lower esophageal sphincter. The sphincter relaxes and the food is refluxed into esophagus. So if you have symptoms of heartburn then check your weight first. If you are overweight, try to lose extra weight. Do regular exercise to reduce weight. Even the

183

slight decrease in weight can improve the condition. So maintain the weight within limits.

☐   Maintain upright posture after meal:

Do not lie down after meal. Sit in upright posture for at least 45 min. while sitting in upright posture the gravity acts on stomach. It increases the rate of gastric emptying and aids the stomach to get rid of its contents. So the chances of regurgitation of food and acid reflux are reduced.

☐   Walk after meal:

It is a good habit to do walk after the meal especially after dinner. Walk increases the gastrointestinal motility and aids the process of digestion. So everyone should adopt this habit to get rid of the acidity.

☐   Avoid exercise immediately after meal:

Avoid any kind of exercise soon after the meal. Give proper time to stomach to empty itself. Exercise after the meal disturbs the gastric emptying and promotes the acid reflux. So wait for few hours before doing exercise.

www.ingramcontent.com/pod-product-compliance
Lightning Source LLC
Chambersburg PA
CBHW071220210326
41597CB00016B/1886